C000318505

the busy woman's home spa book

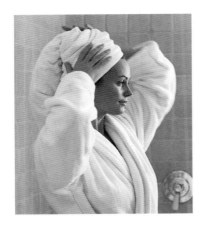

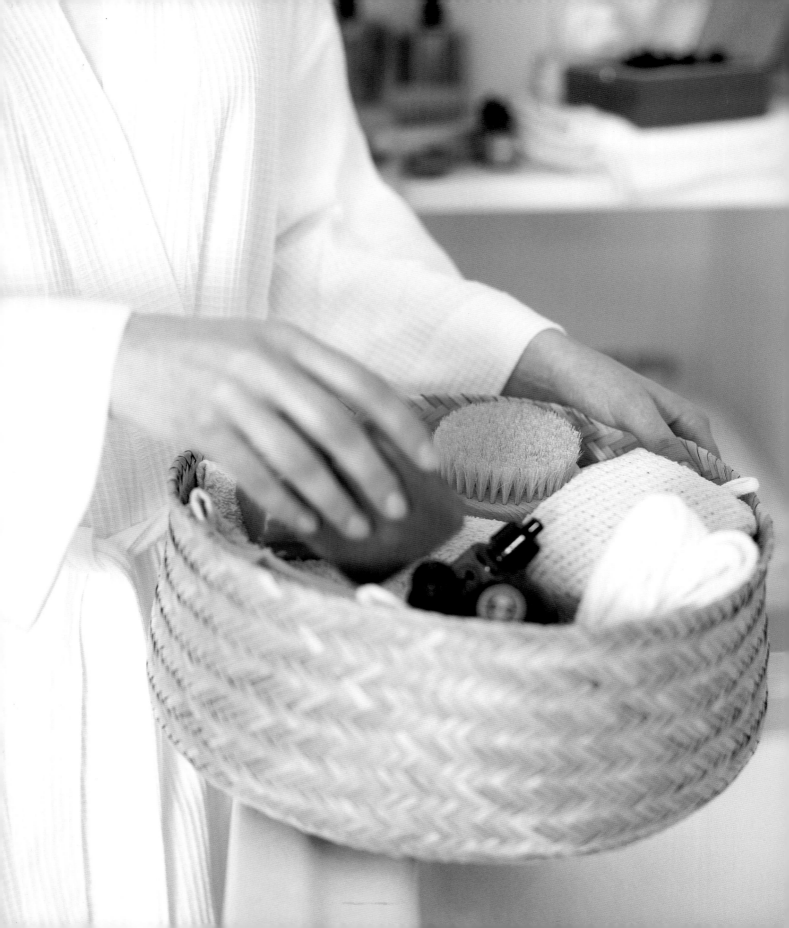

the busy woman's
home spa book

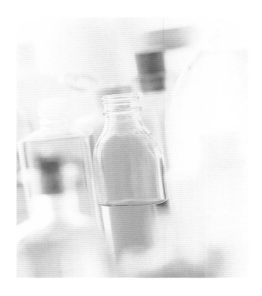

Liz Wilde

with photography by Daniel Farmer

RYLAND
PETERS
& SMALL

LONDON NEW YORK

DESIGNER *Sonya Nathoo*

SENIOR EDITOR *Clare Double*

PICTURE RESEARCH *Tracy Ogino*

PRODUCTION *Sheila Smith*

ART DIRECTOR *Gabriella Le Grazie*

PUBLISHING DIRECTOR *Alison Starling*

ILLUSTRATIONS *Javier Joaquin*

First published in the United States in 2005 by
Ryland Peters & Small
519 Broadway, 5th Floor, New York, NY 10012
www.rylandpeters.com

10 9 8 7 6 5 4 3 2 1

    Library of Congress Cataloging-in-Publication Data
Wilde, Liz.
    The busy woman's home spa book / Liz Wilde ; with
photography by Daniel Farmer.
        p. cm.
    Includes index.
    ISBN 1-84172-974-4
  1. Beauty, Personal. 2. Women--Health and hygiene. I.
Title.
    RA778.W536 2005
    646.7'042--dc22

                                2005005309

Printed and bound in China.

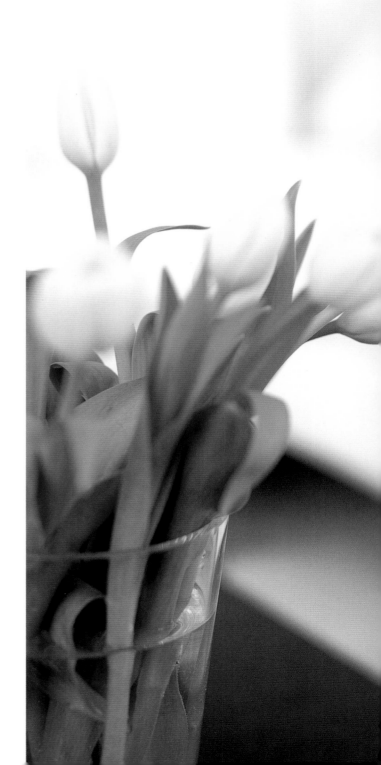

contents

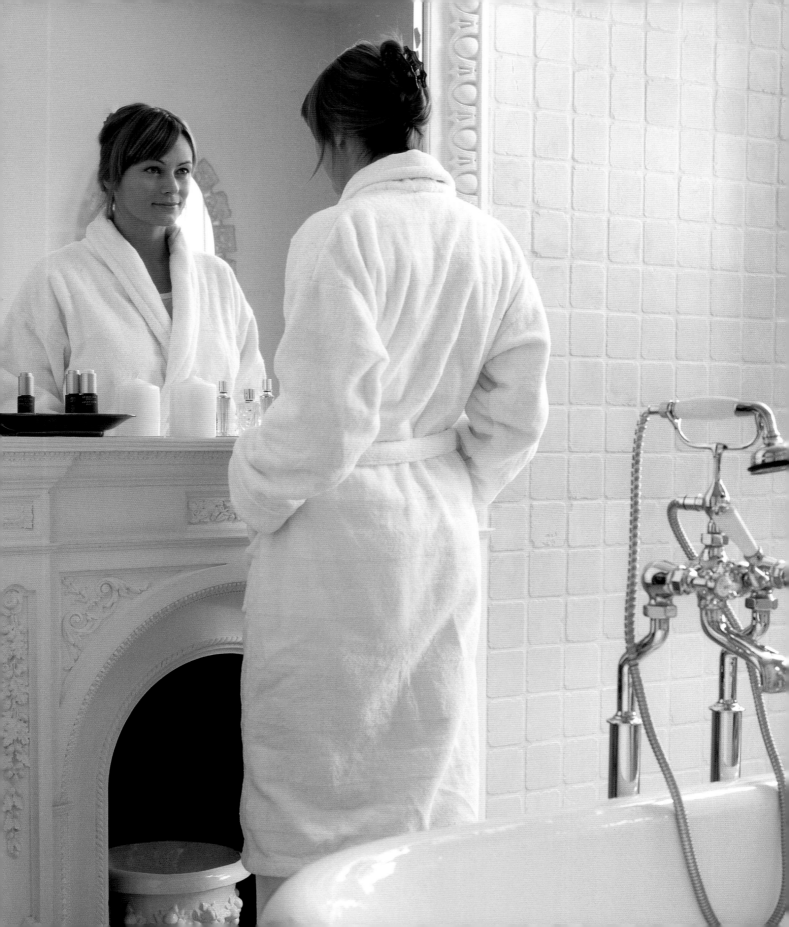

are you too busy to be beautiful?

We all have the same 1,440 minutes in a day we've always had, yet the most common complaint today is that we're all too busy. New technology has been invented to save us time (two-minute e-mails versus ten-minute phone conversations), but rather than using our saved time to do less, we cram even more into our rescued moments.

If time is flying, then you're the pilot. When you're too busy, something has to go—and it's usually you. To illustrate how important you are, hold up your hand. Now, imagine your fingers represent the various parts you play during the day: employee, partner, mother, nursemaid, friend. Your palm represents the real you. If you shut one of your fingers in the car door (while trying to do three things at once, perhaps?), the finger gets a splint, but the rest of your roles can carry on regardless. But imagine if you injure your palm. Suddenly your whole hand is useless, as your palm controls all your fingers.

The most important choice we can make in life is what we make important. Spending time on the things that make us feel good inside and out (rather than setting ourselves a to-do list with no end) is one of the best ways we can create a life we love. And it will not only benefit the way you look and feel about yourself, but the way you interact with everyone else around you.

Spa vacations and day spas have never been so popular. As our lives hit breakneck speed, me-time has never been so precious, and the appeal of spas is that they force us to take a step back. These luxury havens allow you to do little more than relax by the pool between treatments that unknot your shoulders and massage your cares away. Unfortunately, this blissful experience comes at a (high) price, but you can give yourself the gift of free time in your own home every day at little or no cost at all.

To live your best life, you need to be in good health, both mentally and physically. Well-being and happiness are holistic processes. The Greek word *holis* means "whole" and is based on the idea that mind and body have a natural balance reached by paying attention to every area of your life— which means that to look good, you also have to feel good. Improving your well-being feels great, but first you have to decide you're worth looking after.

Years ago, beauty and health were considered two very different things. But as our lives become more frantic, we're looking increasingly toward Eastern healing practices to help us cope with Western stress. We now know that practicing yoga not only eases our bodies of tension, but clears our skin and brightens our eyes. Beauty is an inside job. You can spend a fortune on the most expensive face cream, but if you're still living your life at high speed with no time for yourself, that cream will do little more than sit on your skin as you race through the day.

This book will tell you how to incorporate beauty and self-care rituals into your day, whether you have an hour to spare or just five minutes. From stress-busting facials to stress-relieving stretches. From feel-good food to look-good makeup techniques. Everything in this book is designed to make you look and feel better. There are also lots of easy-to-make home recipes (no more than two ingredients required—guaranteed), so you don't even have to buy new beauty products. And as it's estimated that up to 60 percent of what we put on our skin ends up in the bloodstream, making your own cosmetics is the only way to know what you're absorbing.

Try everything and see what you most enjoy. You need to love these self-care rituals enough to want to spend time boosting your body and mind health every day. We're hard-wired to do things that please us, so the more enjoyable your me-time activities, the more likely you'll stick with them for life.

But what if you're reading this convinced you don't have any spare time for yourself? We may insist we're slaves to our schedules, but we all have more choice than we realize over how we use what time we have. You control your time, not the other way around, so start using it to nurture you, not exhaust you. How many hours this week have you spent on activities that have no meaning to you? Try this simple exercise:

LIST ALL THE WAYS *YOU* MISUSE YOUR TIME

TV watching, e-mail checking, complaining, phone gossiping, net surfing, excessive shopping, worrying…
What could you cut back on? Perhaps you only need to shop once a week?
Check e-mails twice a day? Only watch programs you're interested in?
Start focusing on the good stuff in your life rather than what's not working?

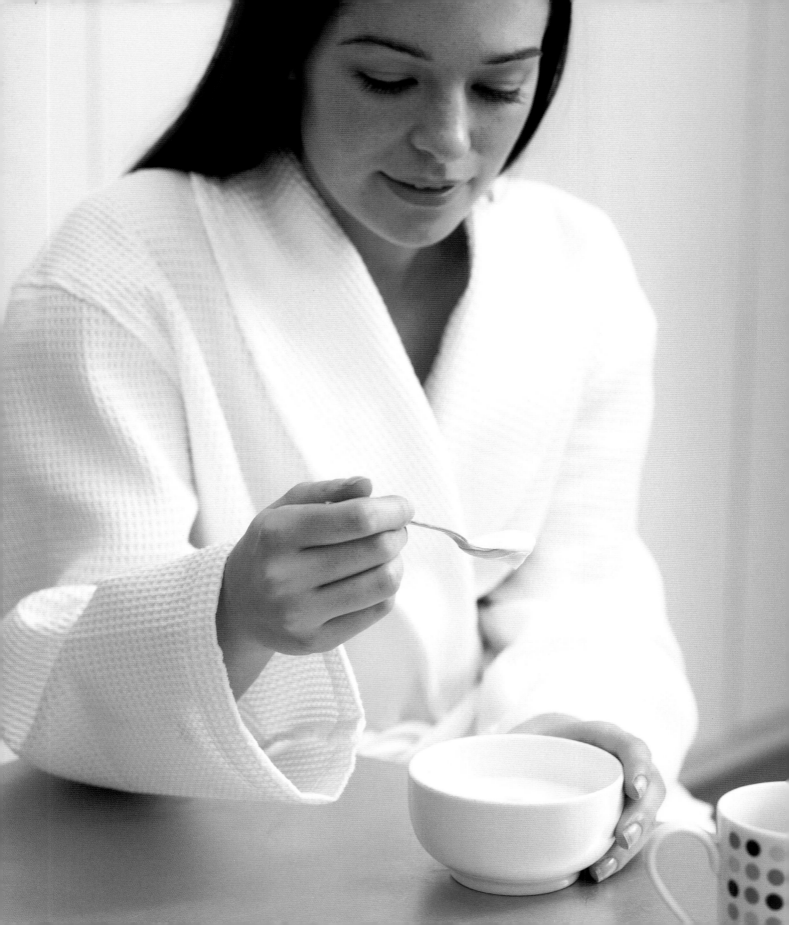

Meetings at work, waiting in traffic, listening to friends' problems, constant interruptions from colleagues, running errands for family members…
What changes need to be made to lighten your load? What can you stop doing? What can you delegate or outsource? Who do you need to say no to? Where do you need to tell the truth?
Now, subtract two things you're currently doing that you don't enjoy, and add two things that will make you look and feel fantastic. It's that simple.

The consequences of constantly racing against the clock include everything from skin problems to low immunity. So if you can't slow down, look at your thoughts. If you believe you can only be successful by being busy, you will always fill your days with tasks and chores. Who said everyone else was more important than you? We live in a culture that tells us relaxing is the equivalent of being lazy, so we cram our lives full of activity. But relaxing is not the same as collapsing—it's simply time to refuel.

It's so much easier to be positive about life when you're looking after yourself—whether that's pampering your face, feeding your body, or simply starting and ending each day doing things that make you look and feel good. So decide today to put aside time for the feel-good habits and rituals in this book. Lifting your spirits works like a natural facelift—the better you look after yourself, the better you look. Isn't it time you started taking *very* good care of yourself?

creating a haven

The most luxurious treatment in the world won't relax your body and unwind your mind if you have to rush for the phone halfway through. To get the best possible results from all your pampering treats and rituals, you need to give yourself a break from the outside world and create a special place in your home.

Your bathroom is perfect as you can lock the door, but if yours is less than luxurious, find another place to pamper and just use the bathroom for its water supply. You'll know you've got the mood right when just walking into your haven makes you feel better. The trick is to indulge your senses for an overall feeling of well-being. Here's what you'll find in top spas, all of which you can copy to bring that feeling of relaxed calm into your own home. Finally, don't rush, and turn off the bell on your phone before you begin.

LIGHTING
This must be subtle to relax your eyes (and mind). Many of us spend our days under fluorescent strip lighting, which can leave you feeling tired and headachy. For the most calming lighting, invest in full-spectrum bulbs that simulate natural daylight. Or go one better—turn off the main light and surround yourself with candles (they also work a treat at hiding outdated bathroom fixtures!).

SOUND
No spa experience is complete without soothing music to ease your mind. Listening to music you love can improve your mood no matter how nasty the day has been. High frequencies stimulate your central nervous system, so choose mellow sounds or go classical.

TEMPERATURE
You want this to be warm and comforting. Too cold and you won't relax, too warm and you'll feel stifled.

SCENT
If you're using a diffuser, pour a little water into the saucer and let it warm up first before adding your favorite oils (the scent will last longer). Or create your own diffusers by adding a few drops of essential oil to small bowls of water and placing them near radiators. Scented candles look luxurious, but you can get the same effect by using plain (much cheaper) ones. Light the wick, allow a puddle of wax to collect around the top, and then carefully sprinkle on a few drops of oil—the melted wax will be the perfect temperature to release the aroma. Scented flowers can also change the mood of a room from practical to pampering (and they feel like a wonderful treat).

COMFORT
Most spas are scattered with cushions for comfortable lounging—an easy effect to imitate. You could also put up photographs of people you love, or objects you've collected that have a special meaning to you. The minute you step into your haven, your memory will respond to the stimulus and go straight back to that happy time, creating an instant feel-good mood.

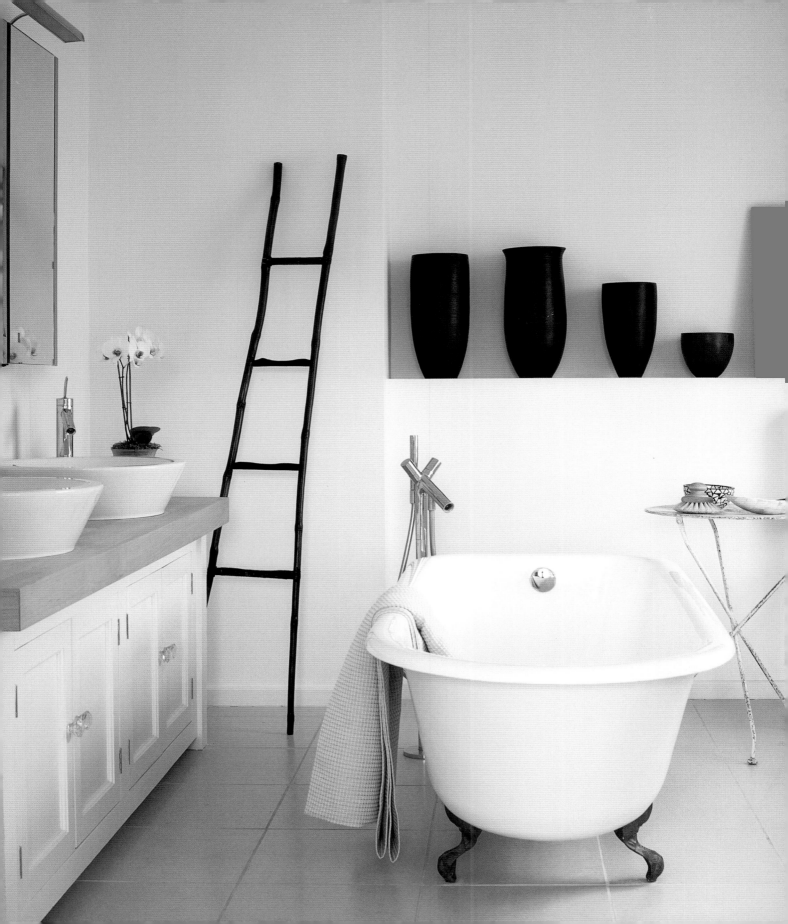

the healing power of color

Color has been used to heal as far back as Egyptian times, when patients would sit in different areas of a room constructed so the sun's rays were broken up into the seven colors of the spectrum. Modern research shows that you can seriously affect your mood by surrounding yourself with the right colors. Here's what a trip to Home Depot could do for you and your haven.

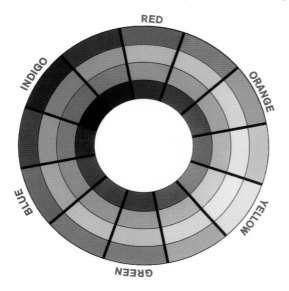

If you combine primary colors (red, yellow, and blue), secondary colors (violet, orange, and green) appear between them. The inner rings show the colors with added white (tints), gray (tones), and black (shades).

COLOR	WHAT IT DOES	WHAT IT HELPS
BLUE	Calms nerves, relaxes and quietens your mind.	Insomnia, depression.
RED	Raises body temperature. Stimulates mental energy.	Aches and pains, poor circulation.
YELLOW	Encourages optimism. Boosts confidence.	Depression, digestive problems.
ORANGE	Inspires joy. Eases loneliness.	Lethargy, detoxing.
GREEN	Aids meditation. Eases anger and frustration.	Exhaustion, headaches.
INDIGO	Stimulates imagination. Promotes optimism.	Weak immune system, negativity.

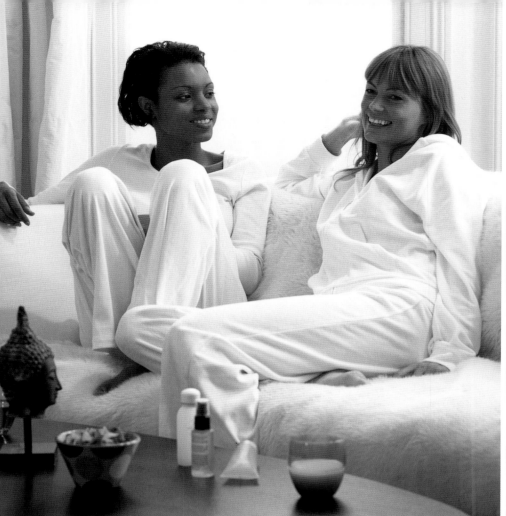
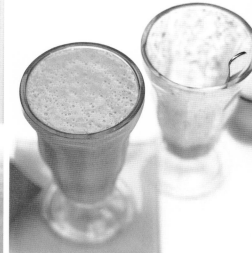
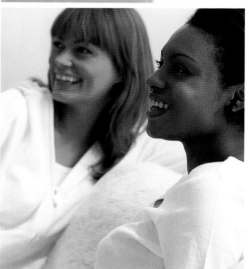

host your own spa party

Once you realize how beneficial the therapies, treatments, and rituals in this book can be, you may want to share them with your friends.

Spa parties are the latest way for the A-list to get together without a complexion-wrecking hangover in the morning. They may go to a $1,000-a-night spa, but you could just as easily host your own spa party at home. Throw a theme-based bash (energy-boosting, detoxing, rejuvenating), or replace the usual wine bar with your living room to celebrate an event (birthday, engagement, promotion). Spa parties work perfectly for any get-together, from a baby shower to a post-vacation photo exchange. Ask each of your friends to bring a homemade or purchased treatment, plus a towel, and bathrobe and slippers if they really want to recreate the spa experience. Whisk up some fresh juice or brew a pot of green tea, and prepare recipes beforehand (keep them in the fridge) for stress-free hosting. After all, isn't that the point?

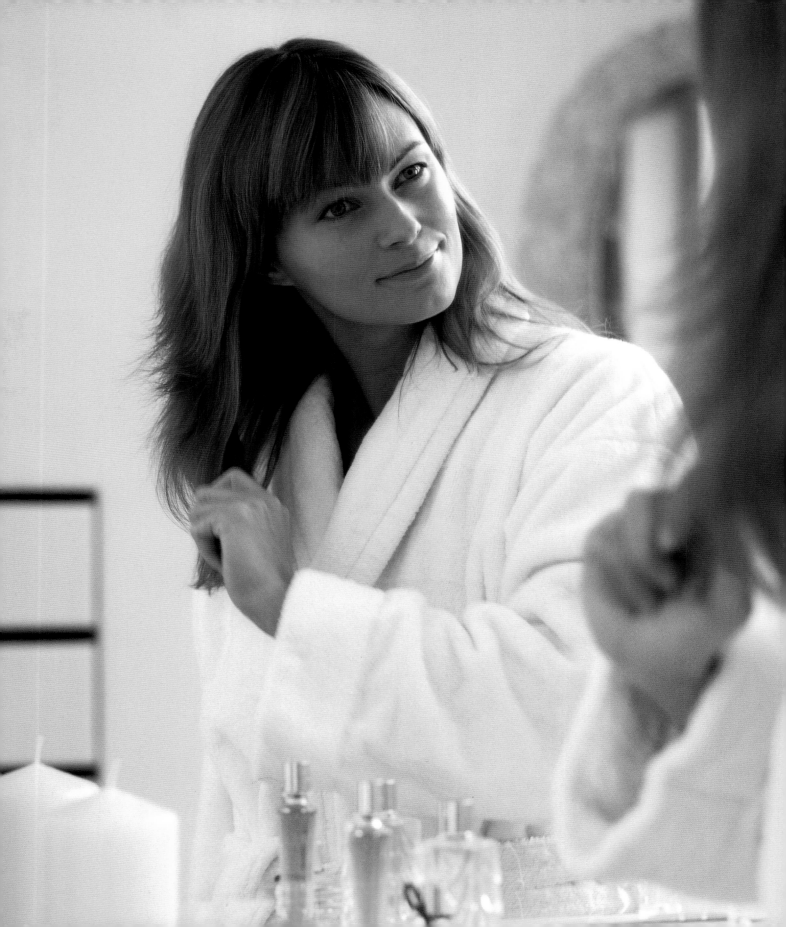

look fabulous

five ways to look better instantly

When you want an instant lift, use these quick tips to improve your looks—starting with the best natural image-booster, a smile.

1 SMILE

Everyone looks better when they're smiling, and a smile also enhances your immunity by improving your mood. Nothing to smile about? At bedtime, list all the things that have made you happy during the day. Most of us are naturally negative, so we have to train ourselves to look on the bright side, but it's worth it. Studies have shown that being optimistic can actually add seven and a half years to your life!

2 IMPROVE YOUR POSTURE

Slouching not only looks unattractive, it causes muscle tension in the neck, shoulders, and back due to the extra effort needed to support the head. It actually takes much less energy to stand up straight with your head held high resting on the top of your spine. Imagine a piece of string pulling you up from the top of your head so your neck, head, and spine are all in a straight line, then relax your shoulders. Congratulations—you've just lost five pounds.

3 LAUGH

Laughter reduces the stress hormones in your body, so you instantly feel less tense. After a good laugh your blood pressure drops, muscle tension decreases, and your breathing slows down—all of which make you look far more relaxed and attractive to others.

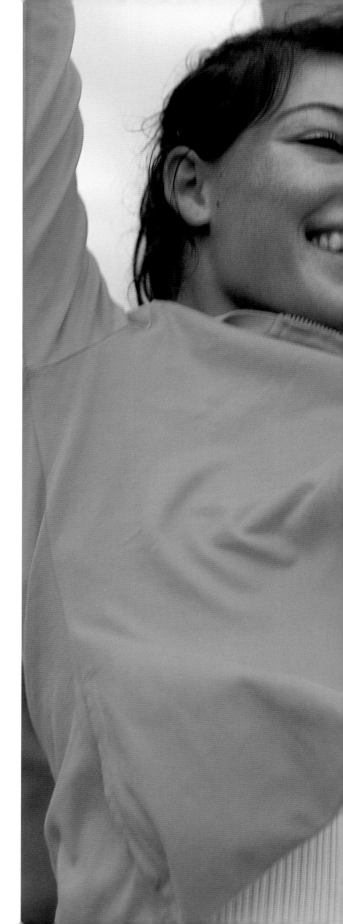

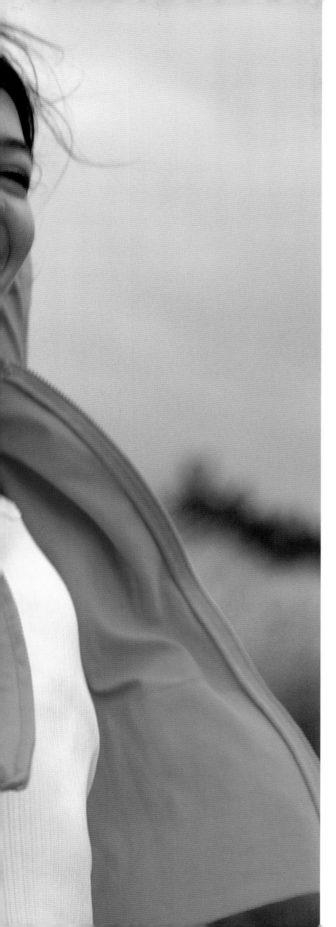

4 MAKE EYE CONTACT

Looking into the other person's eyes for longer than three seconds as you're talking sends out the subconscious sign that you're honest and confident. Plus you're interested in their reaction to you, which is very attractive.

5 TAKE THAT FROWN OFF YOUR FACE

Not only will your forehead be smoother, you'll be healthier, too. Studies have found that being worry-free reduces your levels of a chemical linked to heart disease, diabetes, and cancer. So stop worrying about what you can't control. Worry never solved a problem, and 90 percent of what we worry about never happens anyway—so it's a complete waste of your time.

Everyone looks better when they're smiling, and a smile also enhances your immunity by improving your mood.

six needle-free steps to great skin

There's no need to spend $100 on face cream—or $1,000 on collagen injections—to improve your skin. Here's what any skin specialist will tell you.

1 ALWAYS WEAR A SUNSCREEN

It's estimated that around 80 percent of skin aging is due to sun damage, which means that the majority of wrinkles and other signs of skin aging such as pigmentation don't have to happen at all. The fact is that, far from a tan being healthy, your skin's darkened tone is its immediate reaction to the damage you've just inflicted on it. The good news is that, even after years of sun-worshipping, getting serious about sun protection can significantly improve your skin's condition. So even if baby oil used to be your sunscreen of choice, it's never too late to reach for that factor 15 (at least) and 25 (in hot sun). Reapply regularly to keep the level of protection up. And a word of warning about sunscreens in makeup. Some studies say these sunscreens can all but disappear after a few hours on your face, so always use a separate sunscreen underneath.

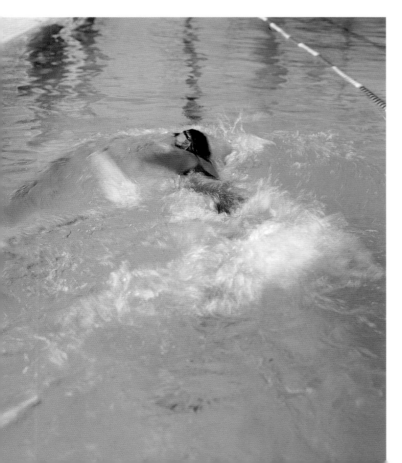

2 GET PLENTY OF SLEEP

You'll not only feel better, you'll look better, too. That's because while you're snoozing your body is working hard to regenerate from the stresses of the day. It does this by secreting growth hormones responsible for restoring cells and rebuilding skin, which is why too many late nights will show up on your face in dark circles and dull-as-ditchwater skin. Fact: if you want to like what you see in the mirror every morning, treat yourself to regular early nights. Many skin experts also recommend you sleep bare-faced so your skin has a chance to rebalance itself during the night. If you have skin problems, you may want to try this, although the initial tightness takes a little getting used to.

3 EXERCISE REGULARLY

Any activity that increases your circulation will bring blood and nutrients to your skin. You don't have to go to aerobics classes; this includes brisk walking, cycling, swimming, yoga, even dancing (and sex).

When your heart rate increases, oxygen surges to every cell in your body, helping each one to grow faster. The result is an increase in collagen production, meaning stronger and smoother skin. Plus, any form of exercise is a proven stress-buster, and we all know what stress can do to your skin. If possible, clean your face before exercise to stop sweat from being blocked in your pores.

4 STOP SMOKING

If the health warnings aren't enough, perhaps vanity will help you kick the habit. The skin of a smoker is likely to look sallow and develop more blackheads than a non-smoker's. Why? Because smoking destroys the vitamin C that keeps the collagen fibers attached to your skin, causing pores to become dilated. Add to this the fact that the skin of a smoker takes longer to heal (the reason some plastic surgeons refuse to operate on smokers), and it's no wonder most skin experts can spot a smoker at twenty paces.

5 EAT WELL

It's no surprise that good nutrition improves your overall appearance, but certain foods are particularly beneficial to your skin. Step forward antioxidants such as healing lycopene, which is even known to reduce sunburn. Find it in watermelon and tomatoes (lycopene is best absorbed when consumed in cooked tomato products, rather than those eaten raw). Carrots and mangos are also a great source of the powerful antioxidant betacarotene, the plant form of vitamin A. When you're at the supermarket, make your shopping basket an intensely colorful one (including dark-green, red, and orange foods) for the best variety of skin-enhancing nutrients. (See over the page for more beauty superfoods.)

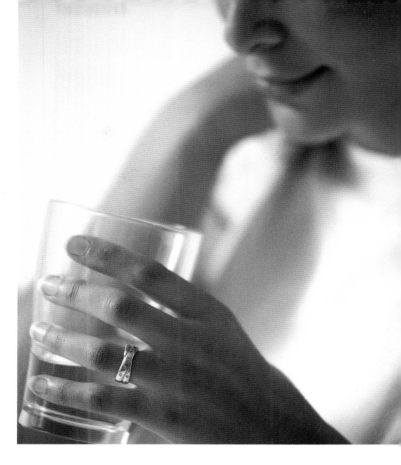

6 DRINK LOTS OF WATER

Water is needed to flush out toxins, hydrate your skin, and help all the nutrients you eat do their job. Many of us are in a permanent state of dehydration without realizing it. A good way to tell if you're not drinking enough fluid (and we don't mean coffee or alcohol) is to check the color of your urine. If it's any darker than pale yellow, you need to step up your intake. Two quarts of water a day will do the job no face cream can, either bottled (which also provides minerals such as calcium, magnesium, and potassium), mixed with fruit juice, or in herbal teas. Remember: by the time you feel thirsty, your body's cells are already in serious need of hydration, so drink little and often during the day. And spray your face with water between cleansing and moisturizing to lock in more moisture (but blot before applying moisturizer, or you'll dilute the benefits).

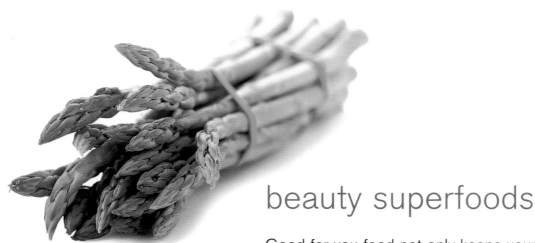

beauty superfoods

Good-for-you food not only keeps your body healthy, it also gives you clear skin, glossy hair, and bright eyes. Here's what the experts agree should be a large part of your life.

FATTY FISH such as salmon, mackerel, and sardines are the best source of essential fatty acids (EFAs, including omega-3), and should be eaten at least three times a week. Our bodies can't produce these naturally, so we depend entirely on our diet to supply them. EFAs are the building blocks of membranes around and within cells, making them vitally important for keeping skin, hair, and nails in good condition.

FRUIT AND VEGETABLES (raw or cooked) contain age-protecting antioxidants and should be eaten every day. If you'd rather not eat a cocktail of unspecified chemicals (and who would?), go for organic, which means no artificial fertilizers, pesticides, or herbicides have been used in crop growing. And choose fresh over canned, as canned versions may contain salt and sugar (if in doubt, look on the label).

GREEN TEA contains some of the most powerful antioxidants available, and its benefits include boosting your immune system and even helping prevent tooth decay. Compounds called polyphenols also protect skin cells by helping eliminate free radicals, and green tea has been linked to skin cell rejuvenation. Not surprisingly, it's the world's second most popular drink.

LIVE NATURAL YOGURT is a great source of protein and calcium, plus its beneficial bacteria help keep your digestive system healthy. Sheep's and goat's milk yogurt is easier to digest than yogurt made from cow's milk. Buy it in small quantities as the levels of friendly bacteria decrease the longer they spend in the fridge.

WATER is the best beautifier around. About two-thirds of our bodies are made up of water, so it's no surprise we need around two quarts a day to keep us topped up. And a hydrated body will have more energy and softer, plumper skin. Drink between meals, or you'll flush away the nutrients in your food, and choose pure still water over (potentially bloating) sparkling every time.

CARBOHYDRATES have had a bad press, but whole-grain versions are bursting with protein, healthy fat, vitamins, and minerals. Whole grain means the nutrients are intact (refined flours have been stripped of healthy germ and bran). Look for the word "whole" when buying bread, rice, oats, and pasta (beware food that's simply a nice brown shade—it could be added food coloring). Why the fuss? These complex carbs are digested slowly in your body to provide plenty of energy, plus the fiber keeps your digestion healthy.

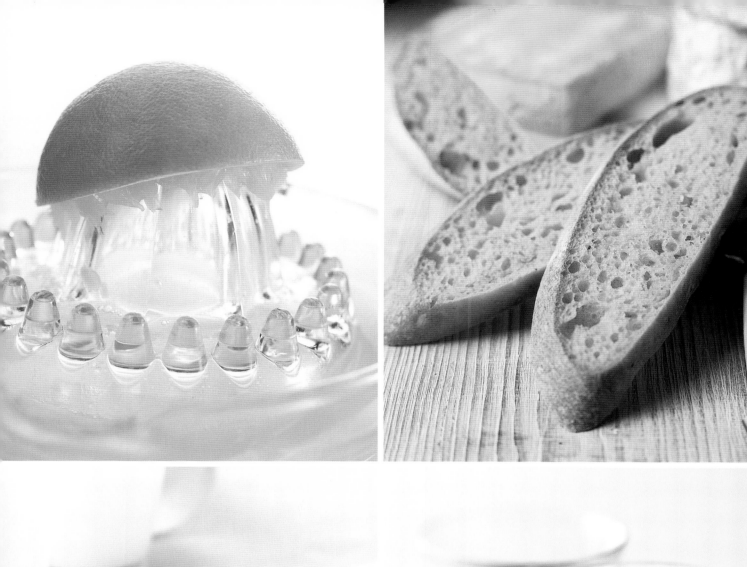
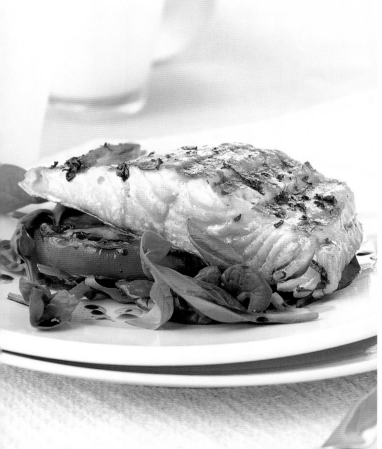
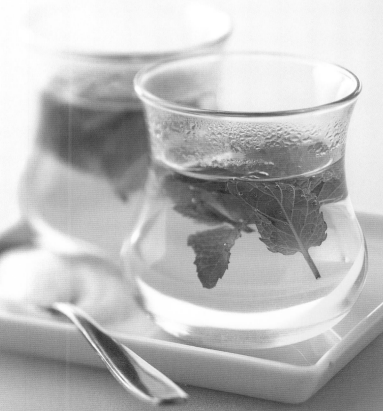

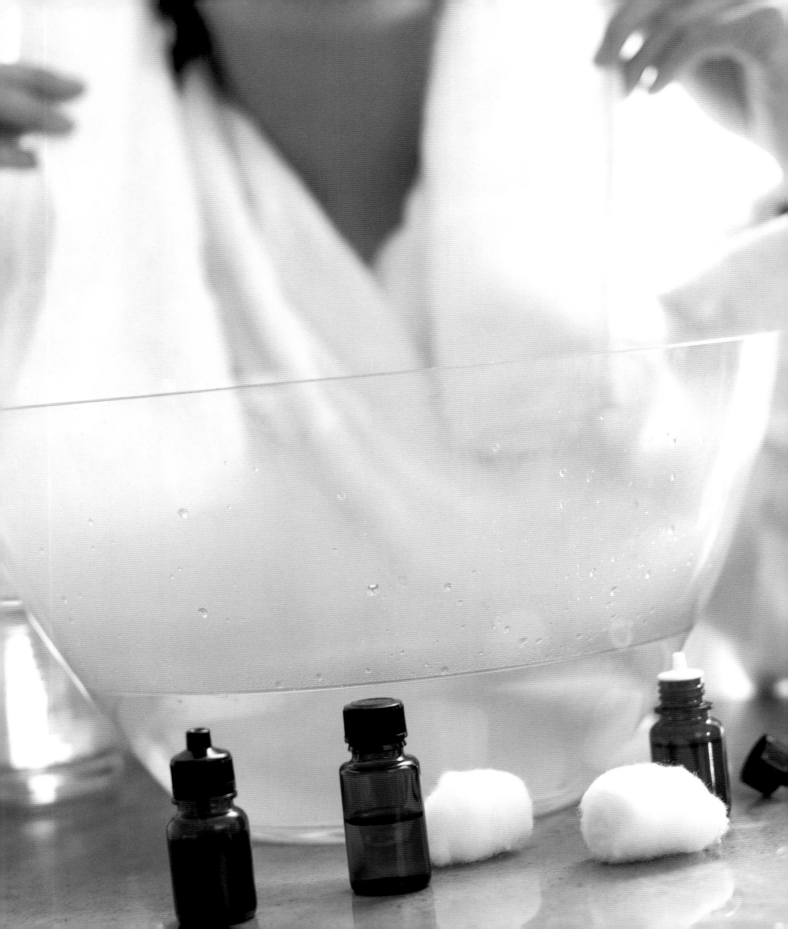

Steaming your face not only opens pores to release impurities missed during your regular cleanse, it also plumps up your skin to soften fine lines. A steam on a bad face day will shrink under-eye puffiness, and added herbs or essential oils in the water will soothe your mind.

treat yourself:

steam facial

I Boil a kettle or pan of water and pour it into a large bowl. Either sprinkle in a handful of dried herbs (use chamomile to soothe and peppermint to stimulate), or add a couple of drops of your favorite essential oil. To decongest sinus passages or ease cold symptoms, use a few drops of eucalyptus essential oil.

2 Let the water cool just a little (you want it to be hot but not scalding), drape a large towel over your head so it traps all the steam, and lean your face over the bowl (at least 8 inches (20 cm) away). Protect the delicate skin around your eyes by first applying a thin film of moisturizer.

3 Stay steaming for ten minutes maximum, taking deep breaths through your nose.

4 Press in any moisture left on your skin with a washcloth, or wipe with a mild toner. Apply a light moisturizer and relax with a cup of green tea, or hot water with a few squirts of lemon added, to complete the detox process.

IF YOU HAVE TEN MINUTES MORE
☐ Follow your steam with a clay-based face mask to draw out the very last impurities left in your warm, open pores.
☐ Treat your hair to a conditioning mask at the same time, as the heat will encourage any product to sink right into the hair shaft.

Warning: Be wary if you suffer from red veins: steaming could make them worse. Limit your steam to five minutes and make the water warm, not hot.

facial exercises

Tight facial muscles can cause everything from headaches and biting problems (teeth clenching or nighttime grinding) to neck pain and facial puffiness. Method Putkisto exercises for the face will retrain these muscles and loosen tension.

Practice the sequence opposite two to three times a week for three or four weeks and you'll see an improvement in skin condition, a disappearing double chin, and brighter eyes. The exercises will also help ease headaches, sinus and biting problems, release upper body tension, and even improve your voice! Before you start, make sure your face and hands are clean, and don't force or strain the facial muscles.

TEST YOUR TENSION
Place your fingertips on your temples and bite, and you'll feel how your biting muscles reach all the way into your hairline at eye level. To test how loose these muscles are, relax your jaw and all the muscles around your mouth. If you can fit three fingers between your teeth, the muscles are in a good condition. Sadly, for many of us our mouths hardly open at all.

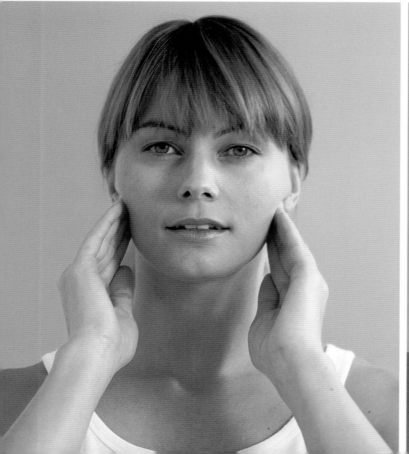
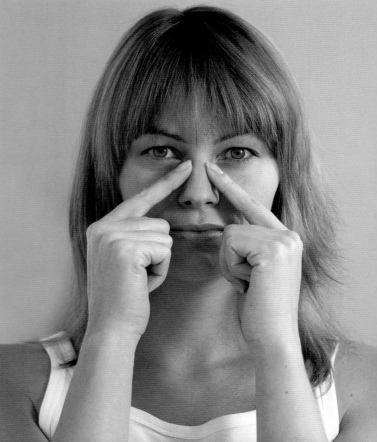

I HORSESHOE MASSAGE

To increase lymph flow, helping remove toxins from your body. Use a very light touch. Beginning at the back of your neck, slide your fingertips around your neck and pause between your collarbones. Press firmly down toward your breastbone. Repeat twice.

2 COOL DOWN YOUR TEMPLES

Refreshes the eyes, relaxes the cheeks and jaw, and eases headaches. Use a firm touch. Place your fingers on the lowest part of your temples. Slide your fingertips straight up, following the temples. At the same time, move your upper jaw and upper lip down, creating a stretch. Repeat 5–8 times.

3 NOSE QUARTET (FOUR PRESSURES)

Centerline Pressure

This will relax the back of the neck. Place the tip of both your middle or index fingers on the inside of your eyebrows. Find this point by following the arch of the browbone, starting from the bridge of your nose. Lift the inside corner of your eyebrows slightly and press. Take your time—count to five.

The next pressures activate muscles around your nose and open the sinuses, making it easier to breathe.
Bridge of the Nose Circle (illustrated near left)
Move your fingertips downward, toward the bridge of your nose. Keep repeating a small circular movement, first pressing toward the bridge of the nose and then releasing. Repeat 5–8 times.

Double Nostril Pressure

Move your fingertips to the tip of your nose, with one finger on each side of your nostrils. Press very firmly toward your upper teeth, count to five, and release. This may feel painful, so relax and keep breathing.

Single Nose Pressure

Place one fingertip directly below your septum, aiming for the point where the nose begins. Press toward the center of your upper lip and count to five.

4 PICK UP YOUR BITING MUSCLES (illustrated far left)

This relaxes the strong biting muscles and releases tension in the neck and back. Place your fingertips on the corner of your jaw and slide them underneath the jawbone. Lift the muscles up and over the corner of the jaw and massage them with a circular movement. Pause, then stretch them by opening the jaw slowly against the muscles underneath your fingertips. Begin from the outer jaw and move toward the center.

5 BRIGHTEN YOUR EYES (TWO PRESSURES)

Both these exercises will increase circulation to the eye muscles, relax your neck, and brighten your eyes.

Teardrop Pressure 1

Using a light touch, place your fingertips underneath your lower eyelid at the point where the lowest part of your eyeball is located, and close your eyes.
□ Breathe slowly and focus on relaxing the muscles around and behind your eyes.
□ Lift the lids gently upward and relax your eyeball against your fingertips. Count to five.
□ Tilt your chin toward your chest and move your fingertips to the outer corners of your lower eyelids.
□ Increasing the pressure slightly, press the eyeball gently inward and relax your eyes even more.

Teardrop Pressure 2

Tilt your chin toward your chest and move your fingertips toward the outer corners of your eyelids. Press gently inward, relax, and breathe normally.

Finish by doing the Horseshoe Massage five times.

relaxing face and neck massage

These simple moves will relax the muscles in your face and neck (not to mention the rest of you), and boost blood circulation to nourish your skin. Tie your hair away and smooth on either a moisturizer or facial oil before you begin.

IF YOU'VE GOT TWO MINUTES

1 Get your circulation going by tapping your face using light, quick movements. Using the pads of your first two fingers, work out along your jawline to each ear, then tap up from the sides of your mouth to your inner eye, and from your nose out along your cheekbones (this also helps blocked sinuses).

2 To finish, tap from the bridge of your nose out across your eyebrows to your temples. Repeat the whole sequence six times.

IF YOU'VE GOT FIVE MINUTES

1 Start at your temples and massage in a counterclockwise direction using the first two fingers of each hand.

2 Beginning just below your eyebrows at the bridge of your nose, use your middle finger to press up slowly and gently along your eyebrows as far as your temples.

3 Using the pads of your first two fingers, tap all around your eyes, working from the bridge of your nose, up and around.

4 Lean your elbows on a table and place your chin in the cup of your hands with your fingers resting on your cheekbones. Starting either side of your nostrils, gently press your cheekbones using your middle finger. Hold each press for 30 seconds and repeat all the way to your ears.

5 Release the tension in your jaw by using the first two fingers of each hand to massage the joint (where the upper and lower jaws meet), in big circles working up toward the ear.

6 Placing your thumb on one side of your throat and your fingers on the other, massage in circular movements up and down.

7 Rest your right elbow in your left hand and, using your hand as support, grasp the muscles all along your left shoulder. Repeat on the other side.

8 Finish by gently pressing your first two fingers just under the bone at the base of your skull either side of your spine. Lean back onto your fingers and then work in gentle circular movements down each side of your neck.

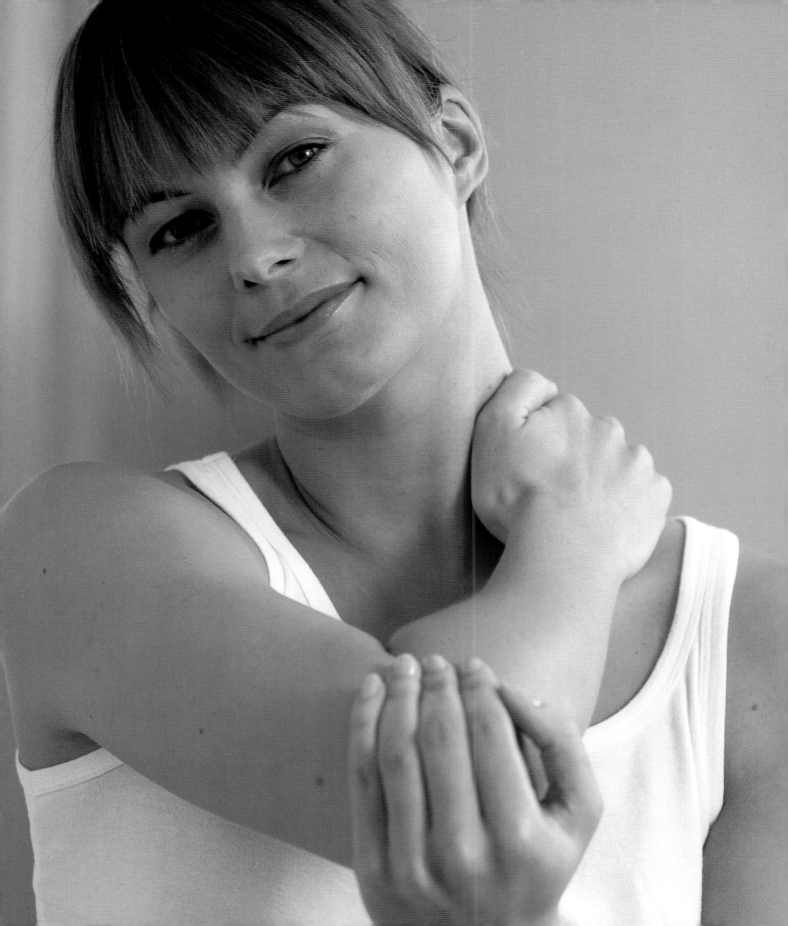

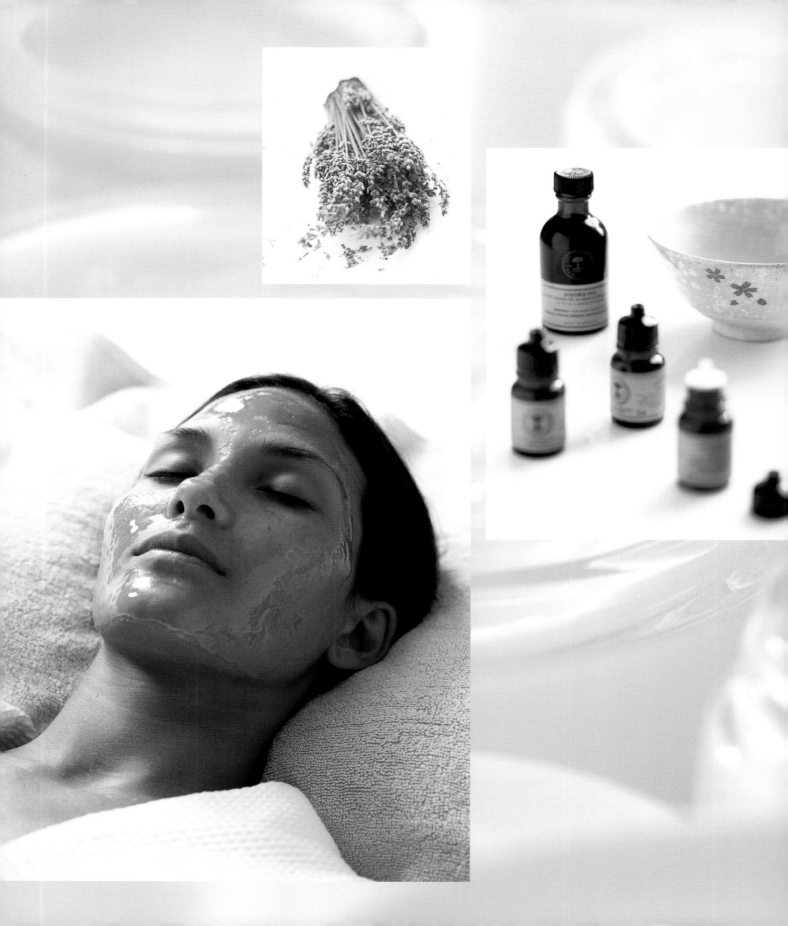

Make your own massage oil for this 30-minute relaxing facial. Pour jojoba, almond, or grapeseed oil into your palm and add one drop of lavender, vetiver, or frankincense oil to aid relaxation.

treat yourself:

de-stress facial

1   Before you begin, prepare your skin by holding a warm cloth to your face. Fill a basin with hot water, add a few drops of lavender essential oil, dunk a washcloth, and wring out before pressing it onto your skin for a few minutes.

2   This massage will take around ten minutes. Repeat the movements three times each, flowing them together, and breathe deeply to inhale the oil's healing aroma.
□ Starting on your chest, work in crisscross movements from shoulder to shoulder.
□ Slide your fingers up your neck and, in one movement, bring them up over your chin, around the bridge of your nose, across your eyebrows, under your eyes and around to finish at your temples.
□ From your jaw, sweep hands up over your cheeks to your ears.
□ To ease tension, sweep across your forehead from side to side, using slightly more pressure. Then, using your first two fingers, use scissor movements across your forehead followed by more outward sweeping to smooth your skin.
□ Hook your middle fingers just underneath your eyebrows either side of the bridge of your nose and press and release all around your eye socket.
□ Drop down so you're now either side of your nostrils, and press and release to unblock sinuses and help you breathe more easily.
□ Finish with the second movement, sweeping from your neck to your temples.

3   Now your skin's ready for a mask. Mature skins love a chopped-up avocado. Leave on for ten minutes or, if time is tight, use the avocado stone to massage the mask into your skin before rinsing with warm water. Sensitive faces love runny honey as it helps bind moisture to the skin. Leave on for ten minutes and relax.

4   After rinsing, pat on moisturizer (don't rub) and do as little as possible!

(easy) natural remedies for tired and puffy eyes

The eye area is the most delicate on your face, as the skin there has few oil glands and so dries up quicker than the rest of you.

USE AN EYE CREAM OR GEL (better for sensitive skin) morning and night as part of your daily routine, patting (not rubbing) around your eye, and for a quick pre-makeup pick-me-up keep one in the fridge.

IF YOU WORK AT A COMPUTER all day, you could buy an anti-glare screen to cut down on dust attracted by static, which can aggravate tired eyes.

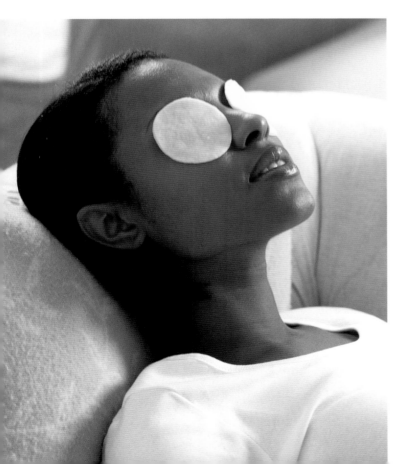

JUST ABOUT ANYTHING COOL will soothe tired eyes and shrink under-eye bags. A couple of cold potato or cucumber slices are the classic solution for irritated eyes, or wrap an ice cube in plastic wrap and stroke over the eye area. Alternatively, keep two stainless-steel spoons in the fridge and place them over your eyes for five minutes at the end of a long day.

CHAMOMILE is soothing and reduces inflammation. Steep two chamomile teabags in boiling water for five minutes, and let them cool right down before placing over your eyes for ten minutes. Or steep a chamomile teabag in boiling water for five minutes, remove and allow the tea to cool before adding half a cup of rosewater (to tone and tighten the skin). Soak two cotton balls in the mixture and place over eyelids for ten minutes. Two chamomile teabags will ease sore eyes after exposure to extreme weather.

THE FATS IN MILK have an anti-inflammatory effect. Soak two cotton balls in a mixture of half cold whole milk and half ice-cold water. Place them over your eyes and lie back for ten minutes.

GREEN TEA contains anti-inflammatory polyphenols which, used cold, reduce swelling, plus green tea is a great wrinkle-fighting antioxidant. Moisten two green teabags with water, chill in the fridge for five minutes, and then place over your eyes for ten.

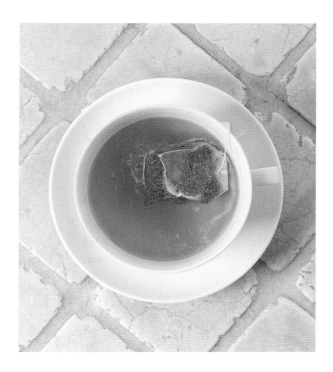

EMERGENCY MEASURES

□ Eye drops that promise to whiten your eyes contain a vasoconstrictor that shrinks the blood vessels, temporarily brightening the whites of your eyes. Use occasionally for instant results on the go, but choose one of the natural solutions opposite for a regular rescue remedy.

□ When all else fails, try a favorite makeup artist's trick. Apply a smudge of silver eyeshadow right at the inner corner of each eye—used on sleepy supermodels by makeup artists everywhere to brighten post-long-haul-flight eyes.

DIY DE-PUFFER MASSAGE

□ Swelling is caused by a buildup of toxins and excess fluid, and you can stimulate your lymphatic system to flush them away. Press gently along your eyebrow and around the eye socket with your middle finger. Then press the point at the inside corners of your brows on each side of your nose, and finish by lightly pressing both your temples.

□ Another quick eye wake-up is to tap lightly all over lids with your first two fingers. Perfect as a midday rescue as you won't smudge your makeup.

Just about anything cool will soothe tired eyes. Cold potato or cucumber slices are the classic solution.

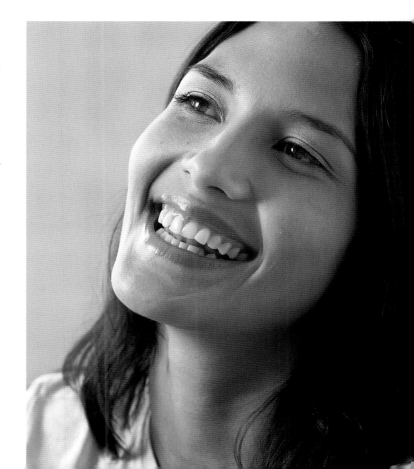

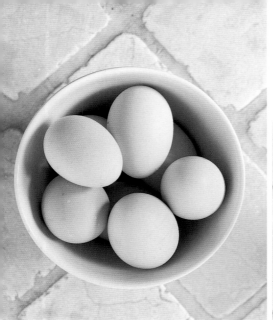
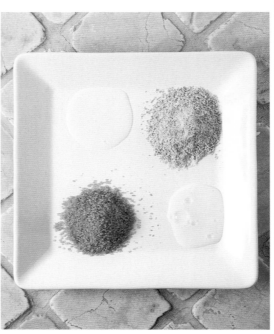
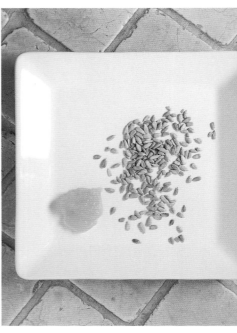

(easy) natural remedies for your face

FACIAL SCRUBS

(Warning: Avoid these if your skin's sensitive.)

□ Make your skin glow by adding a handful of oatmeal or sugar to your usual cleanser and gently massaging it onto your skin in circular movements before rinsing well with warm water. Or add ground brown sugar to warm milk (a natural mild exfoliator), and let the mixture cool to room temperature before massaging it on. Rinse well as before.

□ To scrub greasy skin, mix a handful of sunflower seeds (oil absorbing) with two teaspoons of apple sauce, gently massage onto your skin and leave for five minutes.

MOISTURIZERS

Massage in with sweeping upward strokes.

□ For a nourishing night treat on dry skins, pour two tablespoons of jojoba oil (extra nourishing) into a small lidded jar and add seven drops of your favorite essential oil. Shake well and apply a few drops to your face and neck before bedtime.

□ For a non-greasy, healing treat on problem skins, put two tablespoons of aloe vera gel (antibacterial and anti-inflammatory) in a bowl, and add seven drops of your favorite essential oil. Blend together with a fork and pour into a small lidded jar to use day and night.

Mash one half of an avocado and mix with a dribble of vegetable oil (sunflower and sesame are soothing) before smoothing on.

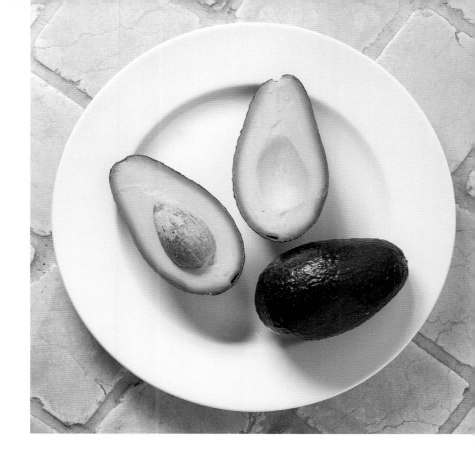

FACE MASKS
(Leave all the following on for five minutes unless otherwise stated.)

▫ Smooth honey onto your neck and face and leave for about 15 minutes until it's dry, then rinse with warm water. Or mash up a ripe banana with honey and leave for 20 minutes (especially good for wrinkles).

▫ Mash one half of an avocado and mix with a dribble of vegetable oil (sunflower and sesame are soothing for sensitive skins) before smoothing on.

▫ Mashed strawberries are great for mopping up greasy skins, while mashed ripe papaya will exfoliate, tone, and tighten. For a moisturizing mask, mash one banana into an egg yolk, spread it over your face, and rinse with lukewarm water.

▫ Natural yogurt contains lactic acid, which works as a gentle exfoliator. Smooth on and rinse off with cool water.

▫ Eat the fruit and use the skins instead. Papaya, watermelon, or banana skins placed over your face will refresh and stimulate dull, dehydrated skin.

▫ To absorb excess oil and remove dead skin cells from greasy skin, mix two teaspoons of natural yogurt with half a teaspoon of cosmetic clay (buy this at health and natural food stores). Apply evenly to your face, avoiding the eye area, and leave for 15 minutes before rinsing with warm water.

▫ Mash up a ripe tomato, smooth over your face, and leave for 15 minutes before rinsing off with warm water (best for oily skins).

The following facial is designed to lift your face and your spirits, using homemade recipes that won't cost you a fortune.

treat yourself:

facelift facial

I Cleanse your skin with cucumber toner, wiped off with cotton. To make, chop up half a cucumber (leave the skin on, but discard the seeds), liquidize in a blender, and pour into a spray bottle to keep in the fridge.

2 Make a face mask with egg white to tighten and firm dull skin. Beat it thoroughly and use your fingers to apply all over your face, avoiding the eye area. Leave for ten minutes to set, and rinse with plenty of lukewarm water.

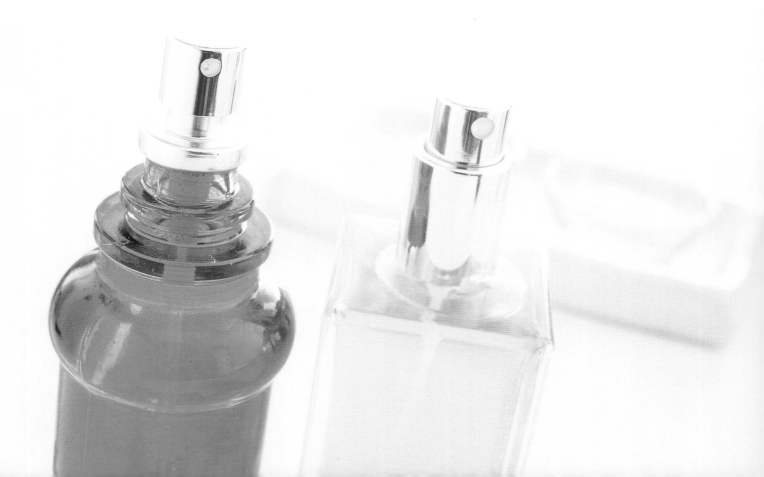

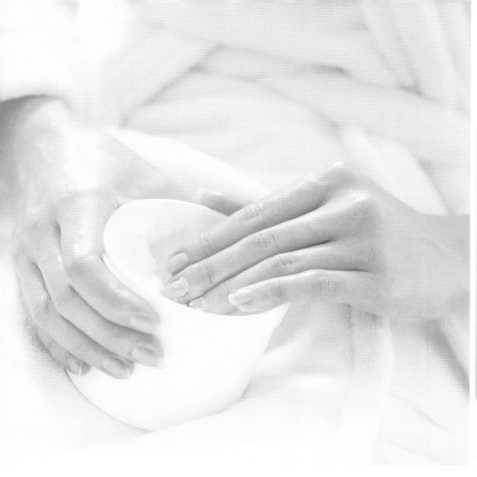

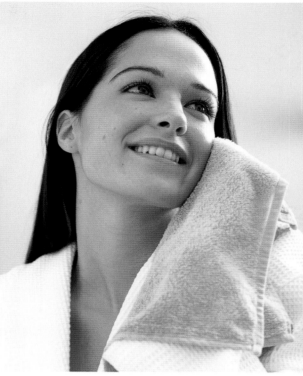

3 Transform a basic moisturizer (aqueous cream works well) into an uplifting treat with essential oils. Scoop into the palm of your hand and add one drop of a citrus oil like lemon or bitter orange. Apply with upward movements to work against gravity and then use your fingertips in quick taps to stimulate your skin. Press around the eyes (avoid near the tear duct as this can cause puffiness), and finish with gentle pinching movements along the jawline, working toward your ears.

4 Leave ten minutes before applying makeup so your skin can absorb moisture.

MORE INSTANT PICK-ME-UPS

☐ Add two tablespoons of runny honey to a pint of warm water and squeeze in the juice of half a lemon. Pour the mixture into an ice cube tray and freeze. On feel-bad mornings wipe a cube over your skin for a nourishing pick-me-up.

☐ Soak a cloth in cold-as-you-can-take-it water and lay it over your face for two minutes. For added zing, add a few drops of peppermint essential oil to the water.

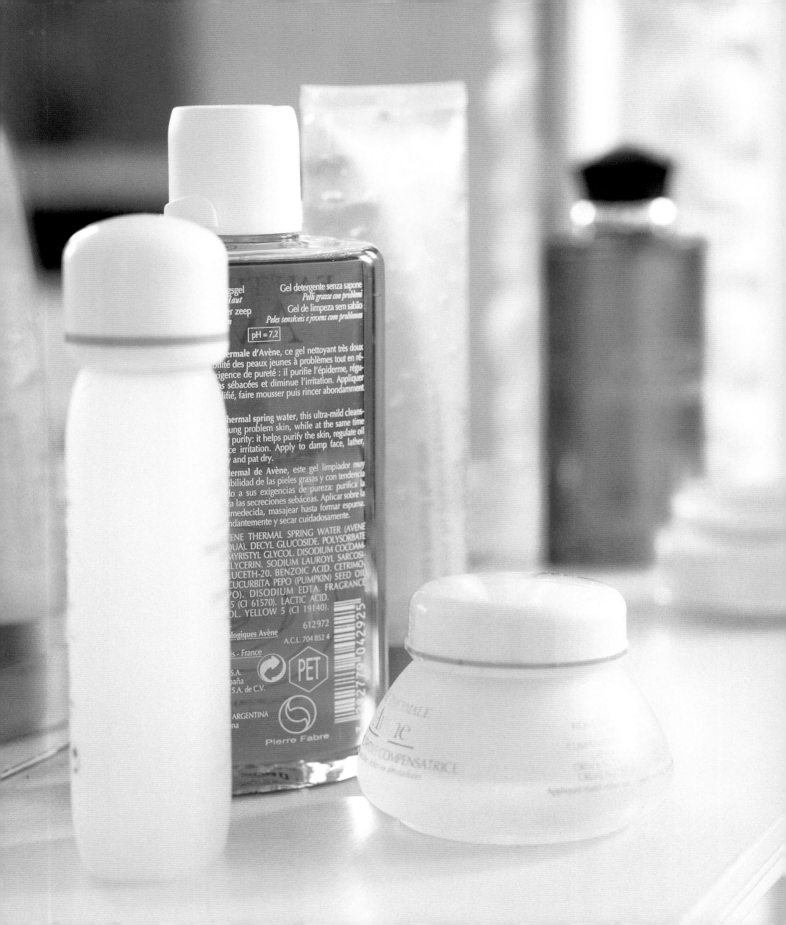

Protect your skin by wearing a
good moisturizer and keep your
environment skin-friendly by
upping the humidity.

busy day skincare solutions

Many skin stresses are caused by doing too much (or the
wrong thing), so you may find you need to cut back on your
routine to help your skin rebalance itself. You can use these
simple solutions every day—no matter how busy you are.

SENSITIVE

Over 60 percent of us believe we have sensitive skin,
and the problem seems to be getting worse. Blame
it on pollution, more complicated skincare ingredients,
lifestyle, or genetics, the golden rule with sensitive
skin is to keep it simple. Which means less time spent
fussing, less heat, less friction, fewer ingredients, and
fewer products. Many sensitive skin problems are
cumulative, meaning you can use the same ingredient
for years, and only then have a sudden reaction
against it. Unfortunately, this often means your skin is
now sensitized, so the reaction will happen every time
you use the ingredient in future.

□ Build up your skin's defenses from within by
drinking two quarts of water a day. Protect it by
wearing a good moisturizer and keep your environment
skin-friendly by upping the humidity in your home and
office (well-watered plants will do the trick).

□ If your skin's being reactive, go back to basics and
introduce extra products one at a time so you can
monitor any problems. Start with a very gentle cotton/
tissue off cleanser and work from there. Take
advantage of tester samples in stores (if you can't
see any, ask) and try a small amount on the corner
of your face or behind your ear. Wait at least 24 hours
to check for any redness or change in skin texture
before buying a big size.

□ Sensitive skins don't like chemical sunscreens, so
look for mineral sunscreen ingredients like zinc oxide
and titanium dioxide, which sit on the surface without
irritation. Other ingredients your skin may not take to
include sodium lauryl/laureth sulfate, petrolatum, and
paraffinum liquidum (a name for mineral oil). Make use
of the ingredients listing to check before you buy. And
remember: even though a product says "allergy
tested," it could still cause you a problem.

OILY

We were once encouraged to use strong antibacterial washes and toners that smelled similar to alcohol. But far from making greasy skins less oily, all they did was strip away surface oil, encouraging skin to make more in compensation. Nowadays, skin experts agree that a gentle approach is best.

▢ Use a gentle foaming cleanser no more than twice a day. Over-cleaning will get those oil glands pumping.

▢ Ditch harsh toner for a splash of lukewarm water or alcohol-free witch hazel or orange flower water.

▢ For a natural degreaser, squeeze a little neat lemon juice onto a cotton ball and wipe over oily areas (just don't go in the sun afterward).

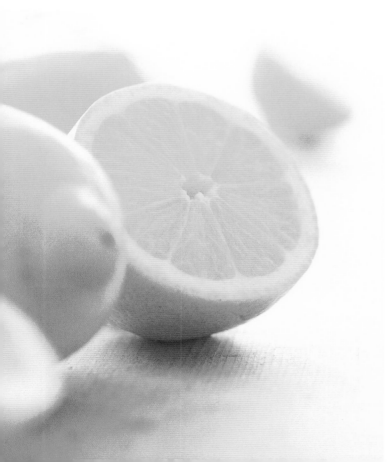

▢ Your skin's best friend is a "non-comedogenic" moisturizer. These are oil-free, so won't block up your pores with more grease, causing potential breakouts. Also look for a non-comedogenic sunscreen, preferably a gel-based formula designed for facial use.

▢ If you regularly get spots in the same place, they could be caused by hormonal changes inside your body (we're three times more likely to suffer skin problems just before a period), or by a bad habit. Common breakout inducers include constantly touching your face (formaldehyde and toluene in some nail polishes—check the label—are also known skin enemies), tucking a dirty phone under your chin, and not cleaning the bridge of your glasses.

DRY/MATURE

As the name suggests, dry skin is low in moisture, making it look thin and papery. Thinner skin shows redness more easily and can feel tight and sore. The obvious answer is to slather on a rich moisturizer, but dry skin benefits from your working on the inside, too.

▢ Omega-3 and -6 fatty acids are essential to moisturize your skin from within. Take them as a supplement or as cold-pressed organic oils poured over salads (much better-tasting than mayonnaise).

▢ As with sensitive skin, keep your atmosphere moist with plenty of misted plants and bowls of water near radiators. And hydrate from the inside with lots of pure, still water. As a rule, for every caffeinated drink, you need to down double its volume in water.

▢ Avoid wash-off foaming cleansers (anything that bubbles contains a detergent), and switch to a creamy one you remove with cotton or a soft cloth.

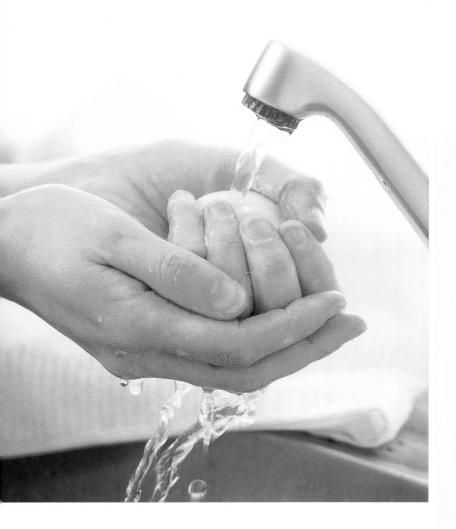

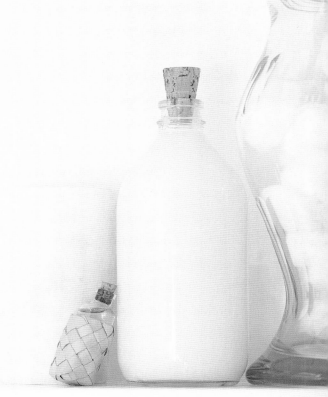

□ Most toners are a no-no for dry or mature skin types, but if you want something to give you that squeaky-clean feeling after cleansing, choose a gentle soothing rosewater toner, or simply splash your face with cool water.

□ Which moisturizer to use? Go by this simple rule. If your skin isn't soft to the touch after you've applied moisturizer, you're not using a rich enough product. Don't be afraid to apply a double helping on your drier areas. Just let the first one sink in before applying the second.

□ Dry skins have more dead skin cells sitting on the surface, so exfoliate regularly (but not more than twice a week). Use gentle circular movements and choose a moisturizing product (for a homemade option, mix a handful of sesame seeds with a scoop of runny honey).

COMBINATION

If you haven't time to use two different products on your face (and who has?), look for skincare that calls itself "balancing," which will take both your skin types into account. Or simply apply less moisturizer on your greasy areas and more on the bits of you that are dry.

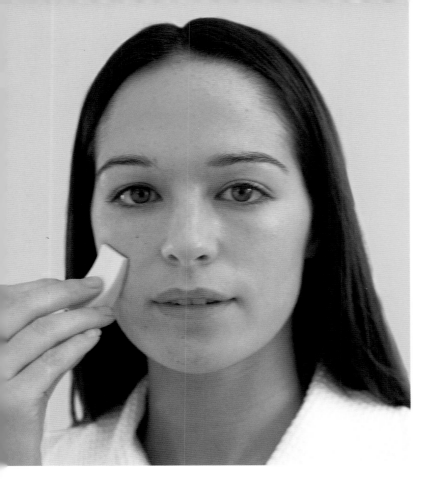

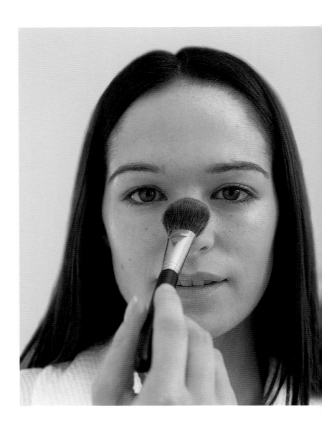

professional makeup lesson

I Foundation or tinted moisturizer always comes before concealer or you end up wiping away your clever camouflage. Apply tinted moisturizer by squeezing a quarter-sized amount into your (clean) palm, and rubbing your hands together before smoothing over your face. Foundation takes a little more work as you want to build the coverage up gradually. Squeeze two drops onto a cosmetic sponge and then press and blend onto your face just where you need it. The harder you press, the more will come out of the sponge, so go easy at first.
EXTRA TIP Don't apply tinted moisturizer or foundation under your eyes, where it will crease, or over your top lip, where it accentuates fine hairs. Also beware of getting color in your eyebrows and hairline—mistakes can be wiped away with a damp cotton swab.

2 Light-reflecting liquid concealers disguise under-eye shadows; cream compacts or sticks camouflage blemishes. Either way, you'll get best results with a brush. For under-eye shadows, apply a tiny amount of liquid where the darkness is (it won't work if you use it all over), and then blend with a brush. For blemishes and broken capillaries, apply cream concealer with a brush and blend by pressing with your middle finger.
EXTRA TIP If your shadows are particularly dark, apply concealer, brush on a little powder, and then apply another layer of concealer just over the darkest area.

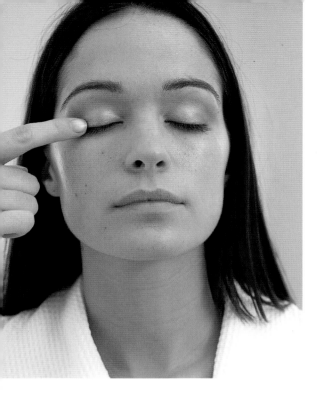

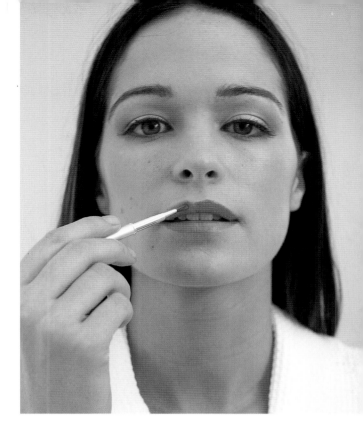

3 Never use powder all over your face. For a natural look, you want a little shine to show through, so just apply with a large brush to the T-zone and any areas where you've worked a camouflage miracle. **EXTRA TIP** If too much shine breaks through, don't apply more powder as the buildup will look caked. Instead, spray your face with water and then blot gently with a tissue.

4 Eyeliner along your top lids will define eyes and make lashes look thicker. This technique may sound tricky, but after a few practice runs you'll be drawing like a pro. Spray a dark powder eyeshadow with a little water and, using a flat-edged brush, look at yourself straight in the mirror and press the brush through your lashes (the line will come out just at the base of your lashes). Start at the outside corner and work along the top lid right into the inner corner. Once the powder dries, it will stay put without smudging.

EXTRA TIP Leaving your lower lid eyeliner-free helps lift the eyes (although kohl along the inner rims looks dramatic for evenings).

5 The easiest and most flattering eyeshadows to wear are liquid to powder formulas. They're foolproof to apply (all over the lid and just into the socket), never look overdone, and dry to give a long-lasting result. Most come with a sponge for two-second application, or you can smooth it on with a finger. **EXTRA TIP** If you're not a fan of color, use a neutral shade to hide any redness on your eyelid.

6 When applying mascara, zigzag the brush as you work up your lashes, as this separates the hairs while coloring them. Concentrate on your outer lashes for the most eye-widening effect. **EXTRA TIP** Avoid mascara on lower lashes as it can drag your eyes down (and end up on your skin later).

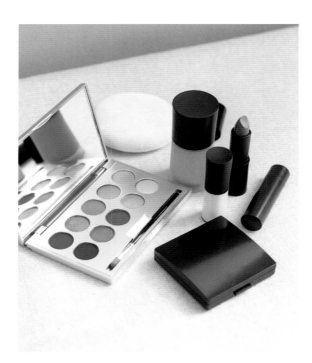

7 Your blusher color should be near your natural color you turn when flushed. Use a large brush and light strokes to apply it over the apples of your cheeks (the fatty part), blending away to your hairline. **EXTRA TIP** Even if you're using a cream blusher, apply with a large brush and you'll find it goes on much more evenly.

8 Whatever lip product you're using, leave lip liner until last, as there's nothing worse than the rest of your color rubbing off, leaving an obvious outline behind. If you're using a lip gloss, apply the gloss first and then line your lips over the top. For lipstick days, first smooth on a lip balm, then apply lipstick over the top with a brush and finally go around the edges with a pencil. **EXTRA TIP** To make your lips stand out or to strengthen a weak lip line, use a fine brush to draw a line of concealer around your whole lip area before blending the edges away.

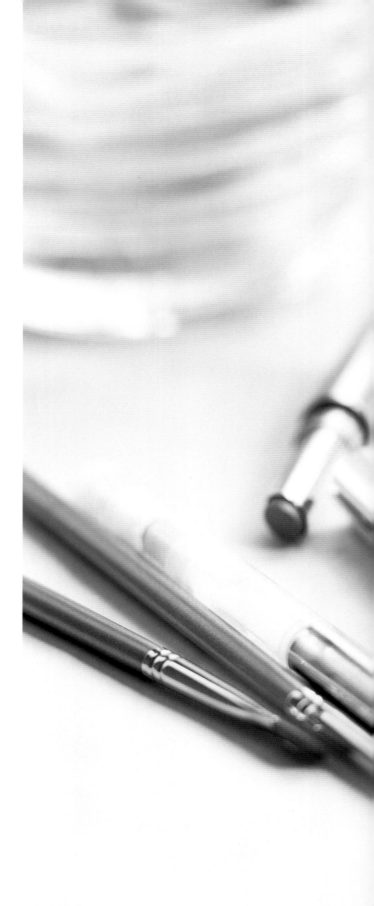

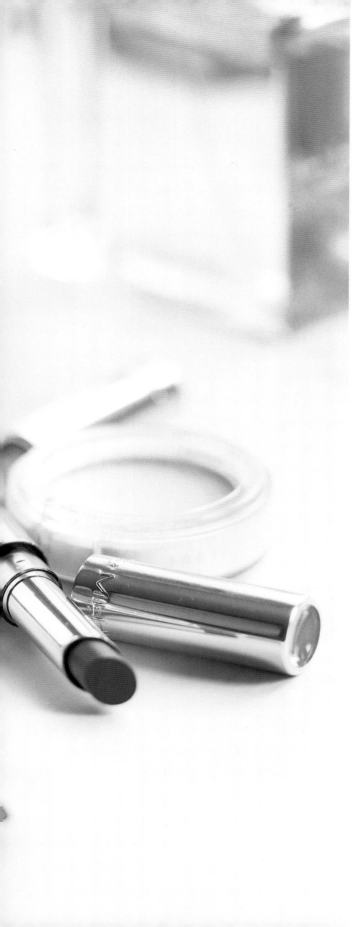

WHAT ANY MAKEUP ARTIST WILL TELL YOU

□ Spend the most on your foundation. You can cut corners on other products, but foundation is worth spending money on. The only way to buy the right color is to test it in natural light, so take a compact mirror with you when foundation shopping. Apply colors to your jawline or just between your eyebrows before nipping outside to look in the mirror. The shade that disappears into your skin is the one to buy.

□ Beauty makeovers in department stores are no longer done by counter staff with little training. In fact, choose a brand known for specializing in makeup, and you'll have your makeover done by a professional makeup artist. Most of these lessons last around 45 minutes and need to be pre-booked (unless you visit at a quiet time). Expect to pay between $25 and $50, which is always redeemable against any products you buy. And there's no need to save your new skills for best. Tell the makeup artist how much time you have in the morning and she can adapt the look to suit.

□ Use brushes for the best results. This may add two minutes to your makeup routine, but adds two hours to your makeup's staying power. Some professionals use a short, fat brush to put on foundation—great for applying exactly where you want it, and no need to wash your hands (or sponge) afterward. Stroke in the direction of hair growth to avoid accentuating them.

□ Most makeup artists wouldn't consider applying their art to an unprepared surface, and use a makeup primer. These clear liquids go on before foundation and after (or instead of) moisturizer. Think of it as applying undercoat to a wall before painting color over the top. The shade goes on better, looks fresher, and lasts longer—and your makeup will, too.

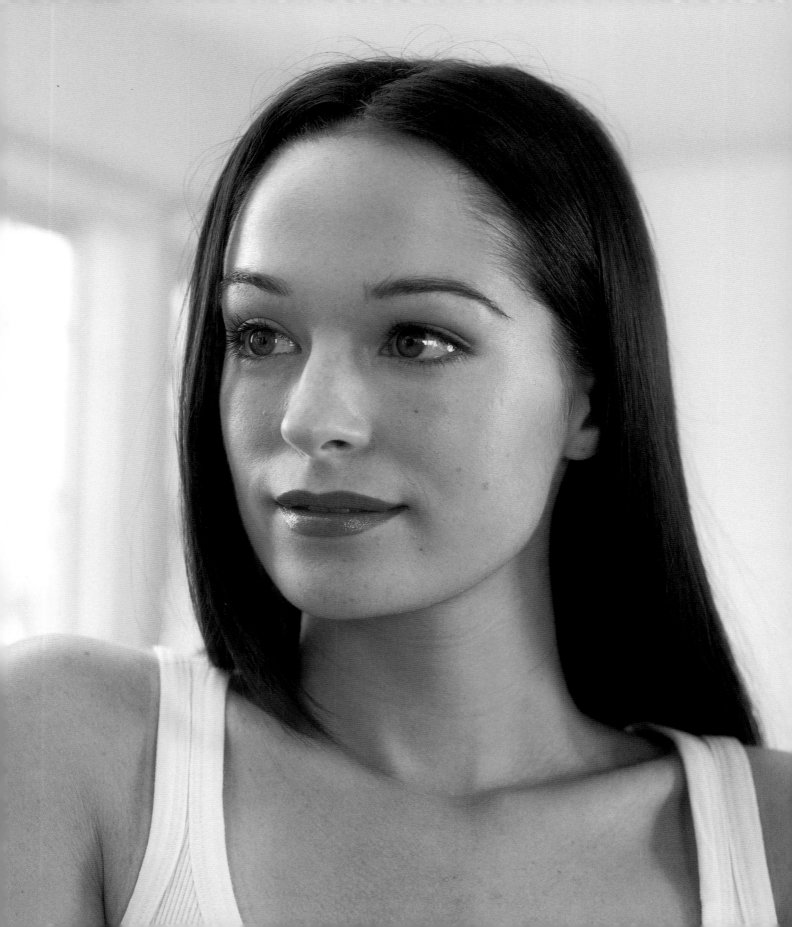

how to look younger by tomorrow

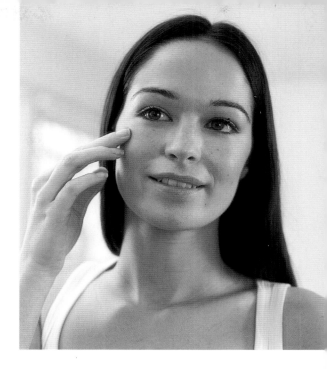

1 A shot of pink blusher can make you look ten years younger. Cream blush is best as it blends well. But don't apply it where you did when you were 18. As we age, our faces lose fatty tissue, meaning it's much more flattering to apply blusher toward the center of your face on the apples of your cheeks rather than along your cheekbones.

2 Eyelash curlers are a must for young-looking eyes. For most flattering results, use the double squeeze method. Before applying mascara, hold the curler close to your upper eyelash roots and squeeze for 5–10 seconds. Release, move the curler halfway along your lashes and squeeze again for five seconds.

3 We lose color from our faces as we age. Too-dark hair emphasizes wrinkles, under-eye shadows, and saggy skin, so consider having highlights or lowlights to lift your overall color a few shades lighter (and perhaps disguise the first signs of gray).

4 Lips lose some fullness with age, but you can create the illusion of it without resorting to collagen. Dot pearly highlighter on the center of your lower lip and just inside the Cupid's bow of your upper lip. Every time the light catches it, your lips will look larger.

5 Get bangs. Most hairdressers agree that bangs are instantly de-aging, but avoid heavy styles, which only suit teenagers. What you want is a longer, feathery fringe that sweeps over any furrows on your forehead, but allows a little flattering light through.

6 Droopy eyelids are a classic sign of aging. To make any droop recede with makeup, hold a mirror at a 45-degree angle below eye level and tilt your head back so you can see the whole eye area. Apply a light eyeshadow shade to the lid and browbone, then using a slanted contour eyeshadow brush, apply a darker shade to the entire crease area in an arc.

7 You can always tell someone's age (even facelifted celebs) by their hands. To plump up weather-beaten skin, slather on hand cream before slipping on your dishwashing gloves, and the warmth of the water will encourage your skin to drink up the moisture. In summer, apply factor 15 sunscreen to the backs of your hands, and hide veins or sun spots with fake tan.

8 Your neck's another age giveaway because the skin there has fewer fat cells than your face, making it prone to dryness. Add constant movement and neglect (how often do you moisturize your neck?), and fine lines are the inevitable result. Get into the habit of including neck and chest in your daily skincare regime, and apply your moisturizer in gravity-defying upward strokes for an instant lifting effect.

what makeup can do for you

Makeup was invented for days when you're looking and feeling less than your best. You can look sunkissed (when you haven't left the office in two weeks) or well rested (when you've been up with a teething baby). The trick, as always, is in the application.

1 To wake up tired skin in seconds, apply blusher on the apples of your cheeks (to find the right place, simply smile at yourself in the mirror) and finish your face with lipstick.

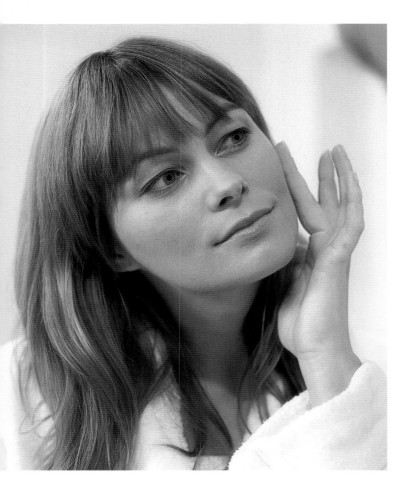

2 Light-reflecting makeup is a lifesaver as it bounces light off your face to minimize imperfections, brighten dark areas, and give your skin an instant glow. Look like you've had eight hours' sleep (when you've only had five) by brushing on a light-reflecting liquid concealer in the following places:

□ under your eyes, blending just along the dark area
□ on either side of the bridge of your nose at the inside corner of your eyes
□ at the outer corners of your eyes over any redness.

3 Get glowing skin on even your dullest days with a complexion enhancer. These creams, lotions, and powders (look for the words "illuminating" or "brightening" in the title) are designed to give the impression of radiant skin. Don't apply all over your face, or the effect will be more greasy than glowing. Just use on the ridge of your browbone, the tops of cheekbones, and along your jawline. Apply with a brush after your foundation or tinted moisturizer and go easy, as a little goes a long way.

4 Get a healthy color with the help of a bronzing powder or gel. To warm up your skin, apply the bronzer just where the sun would naturally hit your face (forehead, nose, temples, cheeks, and chin). But beware of using a bronzer when you're tired, as brown can also drag you down.

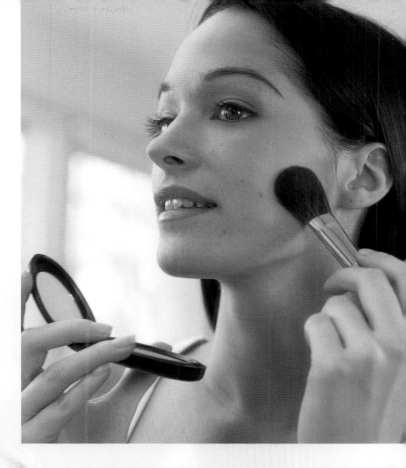

To wake up tired skin in seconds, apply blusher on the apples of your cheeks and finish your face with lipstick.

5 Give yourself instant cheekbones by sweeping bronzing powder just under your cheekbones with a medium-sized brush (suck in your cheeks to find the right spot), followed by a brush of highlighting powder just above.

6 Brighten the whites of your eyes by using a white kohl pencil along the inside rim. But avoid brilliant whites (they look great in pictures, not so natural in real life) and choose an off-white, cream, or slightly blue-white for a softer effect.

7 Make your teeth look whiter with lipstick shades that contrast with yellow. That means avoiding anything with a yellow or orange undertone, such as coral and some browns, and going for colors with a cool tone such as shades of berry and burgundy, plus blue-based reds and pinks.

8 Bring out the color of your eyes by choosing the right eyeshadow shade, and it's not always the one you'd expect. Surprisingly, blue eyeshadow won't bring out the blue in your gray or blue eyes—orangey brown will do that. Warm eggplant shades will enhance the green in hazel eyes, and darker colors are most flattering on light-colored eyes. And steer clear of brown if your eyes are the same shade—what you need is a blue or green to add color.

9 Use bronzing powder to disguise a double chin—apply just under the chin and blend well.

10 Alter the size of your eyes with shading. For small eyes, use a pale shadow all over, with a slightly darker one along the socket line and a dab of white shadow on the browbone to widen. Large eyes suit a darker matte shade on lids, blended into the socket line.

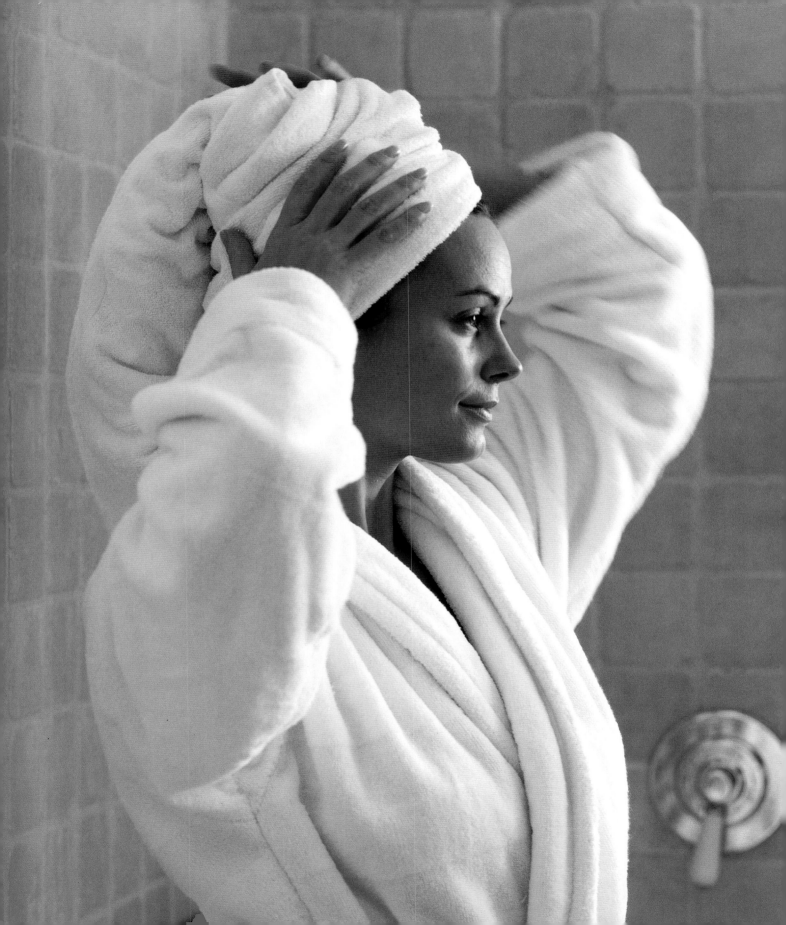

21 (fast) great grooming tips

I Plump and smooth your lips by exfoliating them with a child's toothbrush (more gentle than one made for adults). Twice a week, apply a little lip balm and brush horizontally for a minute. Not only will you slough off dry skin, the brushing will also stimulate blood flow, giving you that just-been-kissed look.

2 Apply fake tan to your face, and your eyes and teeth will look instantly brighter. Moisturize well first, or mix a little of your moisturizer in with the self-tan to make sure the color's diluted for not-too-dark results. Fake aficionados remove earrings first to avoid white marks, and smooth petroleum jelly through brows to stop staining. Avoid dotting the product directly onto your face, or you could end up with brown circles where the tan has grabbed on before you've had a chance to blend. Instead, apply a little tan to your hands, rub your palms together, and smooth over your face in a thin layer.

3 If your fake-tan color develops with streaks, rub them with half a lemon to bleach the brown away.

4 For days when you're feeling pale and gaunt, apply your blusher (any shade of pink will look fresh and natural) over your brows close to your hairline, and then add a little on your browbones to give warmth to your eyes. And don't be scared of applying too much. Professional makeup artists tone down too-bright blusher with a layer of neutral powder over the top. Or you can invest in a lilac-toned powder, which will revive tired, sallow skin. Apply it sparingly over cheeks, chin, nose, and forehead for instant radiance.

5 Remove shine instantly with oil-blotting sheets. Just don't rub. The idea is to press them onto your skin, or they'll remove your makeup, too.

6 Make close-set eyes seem farther apart by dotting concealer onto the inner corners of your lids, extending to the dark shadowy under-eye area on either side of your nose, and blending well.

7 During the night your tongue works like a sponge, holding onto all kinds of bacteria and toxins. Mouthwashes will do a cosmetic job of freshening your breath, but much better is a morning tongue-scraping session to remove all these nasties and make sure your mouth stays fresh all day. You can buy a special tongue scraper from drugstores or simply use a spoon (whatever you use, rinse well before and after).

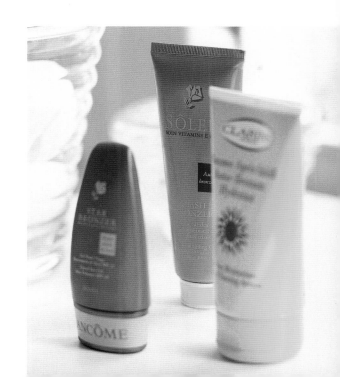

8 When blow-drying, don't make the mistake of trying to style your hair from wet. You're just wasting precious time. Instead, tip your head upside down and ruffle your hair through with your fingers, while rough-drying it approximately 80 percent dry (this also gives great root lift). Turn your head the right way up and start using a brush with your dryer pointing downward to smooth the cuticles on the surface. Hair experts prefer to use nylon bristle brushes, as natural bristles can cause static and make your hair fly away. Style the front of your hair first as that's what everyone sees (plus it dries fastest), and then carry on working through the sides and back if you've got time. Finally, finish with a quick blast of cold air to set your style.

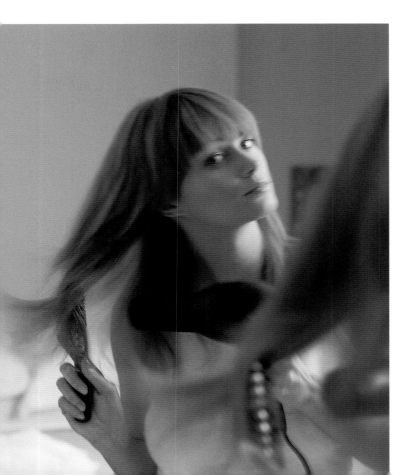

9 Stop lipstick from getting on your teeth by following this model's tip. Pucker up as if you're about to give someone a kiss, then pop your first finger in your mouth and pull it out again. Any excess color on the inside of your lips will come off on your finger, not in 20 minutes on your teeth.

10 Never use a pencil to emphasize your brows—powder gives a much more natural finish. Invest in a stiff, angled eyebrow brush and, starting at the inside corner working out, use light strokes to deposit the color on the eyebrow hairs rather than the skin itself.

11 Groomed brows smarten up your whole face, and accentuating the natural arch also gives your eyes a natural lift. The highest point of each brow should line up with the outer edge of your iris, and the most flattering brows start just above the inner corner of the eye, extending as far as possible at the outer edges. Tweeze after a bath or shower when your pores are open, or dab on some teething or mouth ulcer gel to numb the area. It's a myth that you can only pluck from underneath—stray hairs on top of your brows look just as messy. But go slowly, as brows grow back less quickly than other body hair (expect to wait six weeks before you can try again).

12 Use a clean mascara wand (wipe a finished one in eye makeup remover, wash and dry) to brush brows up and along. Or invest in clear mascara to set your just-groomed brows in place.

13 There's no substitute for a good trim, but when heated styling tools or home colorants have left you with split ends, try this quick-fix trick. Take a section of hair, twist it tightly so all the little ends stick out, and snip off the split ones with sharp scissors.

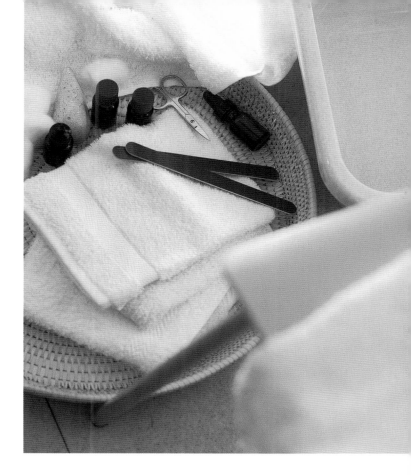

14 Stuck without your full makeup kit? Then get creative. A little blusher or pinky/purple eyeshadow can do the work of lipstick. Brush on and then seal with a coat of lip balm. And if you're caught short with a spot and no concealer, the residue around the top of your foundation bottle is the perfect consistency for covering blemishes, and exactly the right skin tone to go totally unnoticed.

15 Make facial hair invisible with bleach. Invest in a home-bleaching kit especially formulated for the face and leave the mixture on for ten minutes before rinsing (do a patch test first to check for sensitivity). Not only will your hairs look less obvious, the bleach will soften their texture, too.

16 Before waxing, be kind to yourself by placing a warm washcloth on the area to open the pores and reduce pain. Smooth on the strip and, taking a deep breath, hold the skin taut (the secret of getting all the hairs in one swipe), and pull off fast as you breathe out. Regular waxing will make the regrowth finer and eventually actually stop hair from growing, so at least you won't have to do it forever.

17 Make the most of a less-than-ample cleavage with a good bra and a little clever shading. Choose a natural matte blusher that's not too far from your own skin tone and apply with a large brush between your breasts in a curved Y shape. Follow with a little highlighter along the top of your breasts to emphasize their (bra-enhanced) fullness.

18 For an instant skin soother, drench a cotton pad in rosewater and swipe it over your face a few times. Orange flower water works well too, and is perfect for super-sensitive skins.

19 No time to wait around for nail polish to dry (and who has)? Then buff your nails to a healthy pink shine instead, using a buffing file. The friction of buffing also stimulates blood flow, encouraging nails to grow faster. A word of warning: Never buff without first applying a nail oil or cream. Without it, buffing can literally take the top layer off your nails, weakening them in double-quick time. Simply smooth on your product and buff in a sideways motion for 30 seconds a nail (no longer).

20 The best time to push back your cuticles is straight after a bath or shower, when the skin is soft. The quickest method? Use the pointed edge of a towel. Two minutes tops.

21 Every time you apply lip balm, rub a little into your cuticles to keep them soft and pliable.

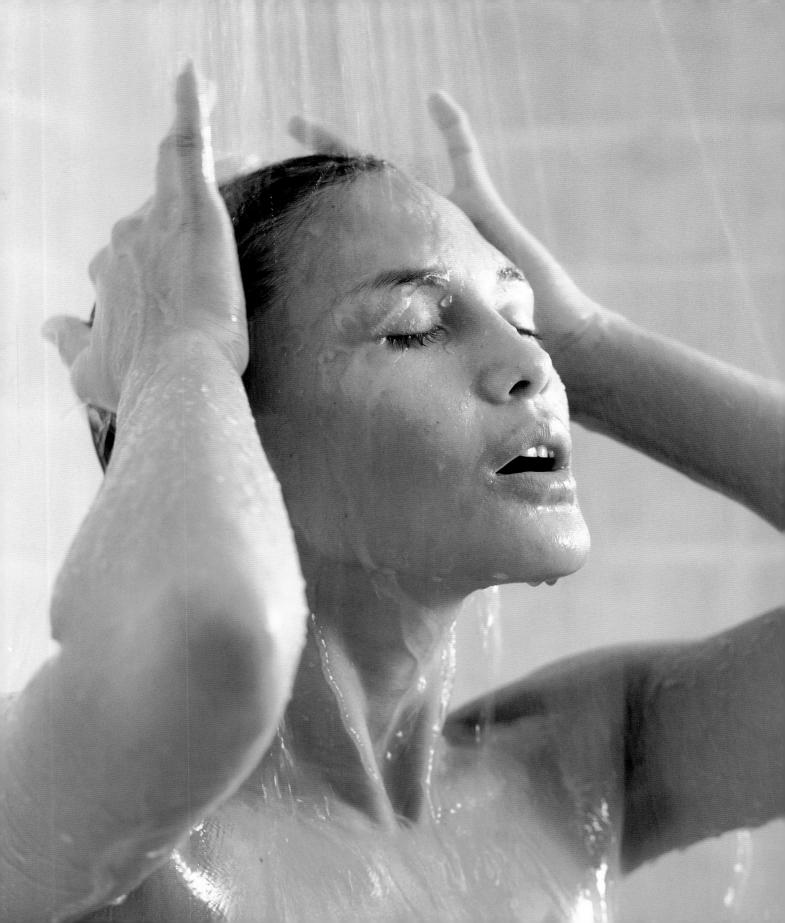

(easy) natural remedies for your hair

CONDITIONERS

Heat-styling sessions and sun exposure damage hair. Little wonder the cuticles on the surface are left sticking out in all directions, resulting in dull-looking hair as the outer layer no longer reflects light. Combing through one of these deep conditioners (with a wide-tooth comb) will smooth the surface so light can bounce off it again. Treat your hair weekly if it's damaged, or two-weekly if you have normal hair, and leave it to dry naturally as often as possible.

□ Mayonnaise is the perfect conditioner for dry hair. Smooth on, massage in, and then cover your head with plastic wrap to encourage the mayonnaise to sink in. Rinse off with lukewarm water to avoid curdling. For more heavy-duty moisturizing, mix mayonnaise with half an avocado and massage into hair. Cover your head and leave for 20 minutes before rinsing. Follow with one shampoo and condition as normal.

□ Olive oil is the classic deep treatment for dehydrated hair. Massage two teaspoons of oil over your hair and cover with a lightweight shower cap (the sort you find in hotel bathrooms). Leave overnight for extra-soft results, or for 20–30 minutes. To remove, apply shampoo before rinsing, then shampoo again as normal. You can make this treatment extra luxurious by adding 3–4 drops of your favorite essential oil.

□ Mash together half a banana with two tablespoons of coconut milk. Massage through your hair and leave for ten minutes before washing off with lukewarm water.

NATURAL RINSES

□ To remove styling product buildup from dull hair, add half a cup of white vinegar to a jug of boiling water, let it cool, and use as a second (lather-free) shampoo.

□ Use mint tea as a final rinse to give greasy hair shine.

□ One tablespoon of vinegar in a pint of warm water will ease tangles in dry and chemically treated hair.

□ Give limp hair volume by using cola as a final rinse.

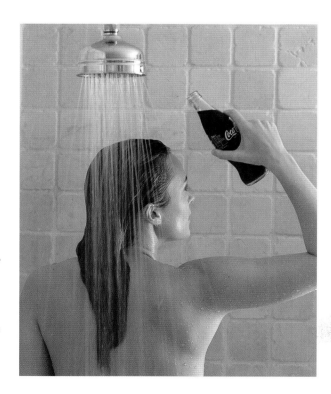

body and mind cleansing

Both showers and baths are seriously therapeutic. In a shower, the water on your skin gives the same feeling as a massage, while a bath makes you feel cocooned due to being weightless in the warm water.

Ever wondered why a long, luxurious bath is all you can think about after a hard day? That's because, just like flotation, bathing also has a beneficial effect on the neurochemicals in your brain, encouraging the release of feel-good endorphins. The result is an almost instant reduction in stress levels.

Showering has a similar restorative effect, as cleansing your body can literally feel like you're scrubbing off the stresses of the day. When we feel clean on the outside, we're more likely to feel clean on the inside—think of it as washing your cares down the drain.

Bathing rituals have been a part of pampering since ancient times (remember Cleopatra and her modesty-preserving milk bath?). What they knew even back then was that bathing can be so much more than just skin washing. Add your favorite essential oils to the water, and it turns into a healing experience for both mind and body. See opposite for some essential oil suggestions.

Used in conjunction with warm water, the therapeutic benefits of essential oils are increased, because heat encourages capillaries to come to the surface of your skin so the oil can be absorbed straight into your bloodstream. Add no more than six drops in total and soak for 20 minutes (any longer and you'll dehydrate and emerge prunelike). Don't make the water too hot; 97–100°F (36–38°C) is ideal. Add the oils after your bath water has run so the vapors don't escape in the steam. Sprinkle oils at the faucet end and agitate the water well before stepping in, as some essential oils (especially citrus) may sting the skin if they are not properly dispersed.

You can also benefit from essential oils in your shower. Simply sprinkle six drops over the shower floor, and as the warm water hits they'll disperse and diffuse into the steam.

See pages 66–67 for more natural bath additives.

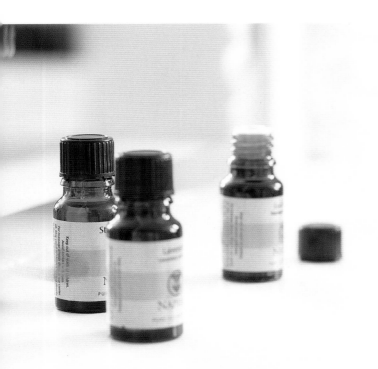

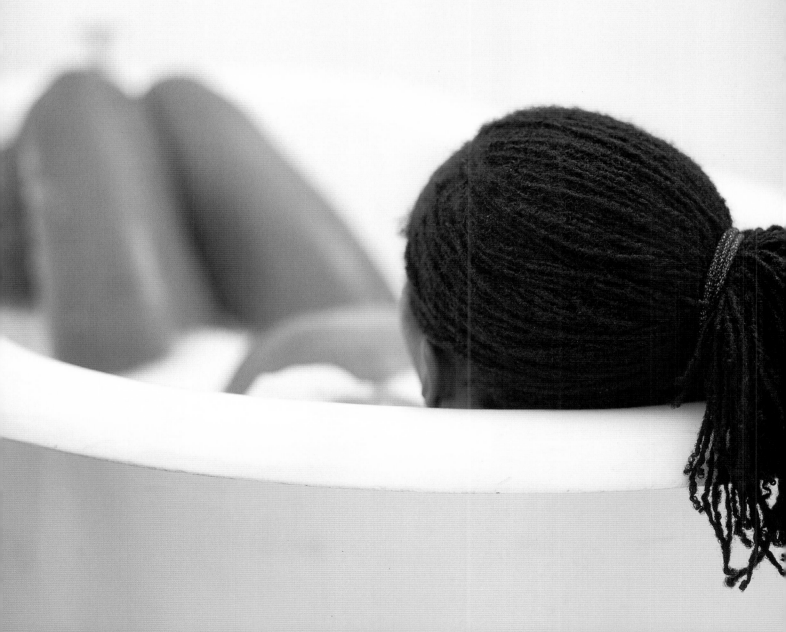

Ten Top Oils For Relaxing

Chamomile · Lavender · Neroli · Rose · Mandarin · Vetivert
Sweet Marjoram · Clary Sage · Frankincense · Lemongrass

Ten Top Oils For Energizing

Grapefruit · Bergamot · Eucalyptus · Orange · Peppermint
Juniper · Fennel · Rosemary · Geranium · Lemon

water therapy

Water therapy has been used to cure health problems since ancient Greek, Roman, and Celtic times. Now popular in spas everywhere, it's easy (and free) to do yourself at home.

A FREEZING COLD SHOWER is the best way to start your day, as it will instantly wake you up and stimulate every part of your body—including your brain. Stay under for 30 seconds to one minute before switching the dial back to warm.

TRY HOME THERMOTHERAPY by alternating warm water with cold for 30 seconds each. Cold on the body sends blood to your organs, while warm brings it rushing back to the muscles, adding up to a serious boost for your circulation and immune system.

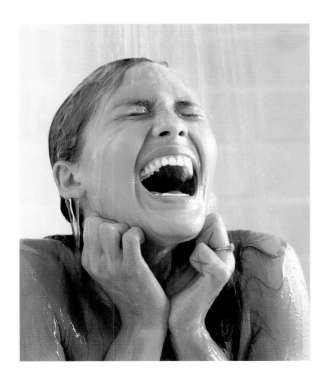

TO BRIGHTEN A TIRED COMPLEXION aim a gentle cold shower at your face, working in circular movements, and pat dry with your hands.

IMPROVE THE APPEARANCE OF CELLULITE by using a high-pressure shower head on your legs and bottom. Work toward the heart to encourage toxin drainage.

TRY A LITTLE REFLEXOLOGY Lie back in warm water with two tennis balls resting on the end of the bath under your feet. Rotate them, gripping and releasing with your toes to stimulate nerve endings in your feet. With 72,000 per foot, you're guaranteed to hit the spot.

THALASSOTHERAPY is spa treatments using sea water and seaweed. Minerals present in sea water are similar to those in the body, meaning they are easy to absorb through your skin. Benefits include increased energy and better circulation. Invest in a sea bath product (see page 124) and follow this five-step treatment:
1 Relax in a not-too-hot bath (the minerals and trace elements in your sea product will raise the temperature a few degrees for extra penetration).
2 Shower without soap to leave maximum minerals on your skin (only half have been absorbed so far).
3 Rest for 20 minutes wrapped in a terrycloth robe so the remaining trace elements can sink in.
4 Shower with soap to remove any bath residue.
5 Grit your teeth and turn the water to cold, as this tightens pores and locks in the treatment benefits.

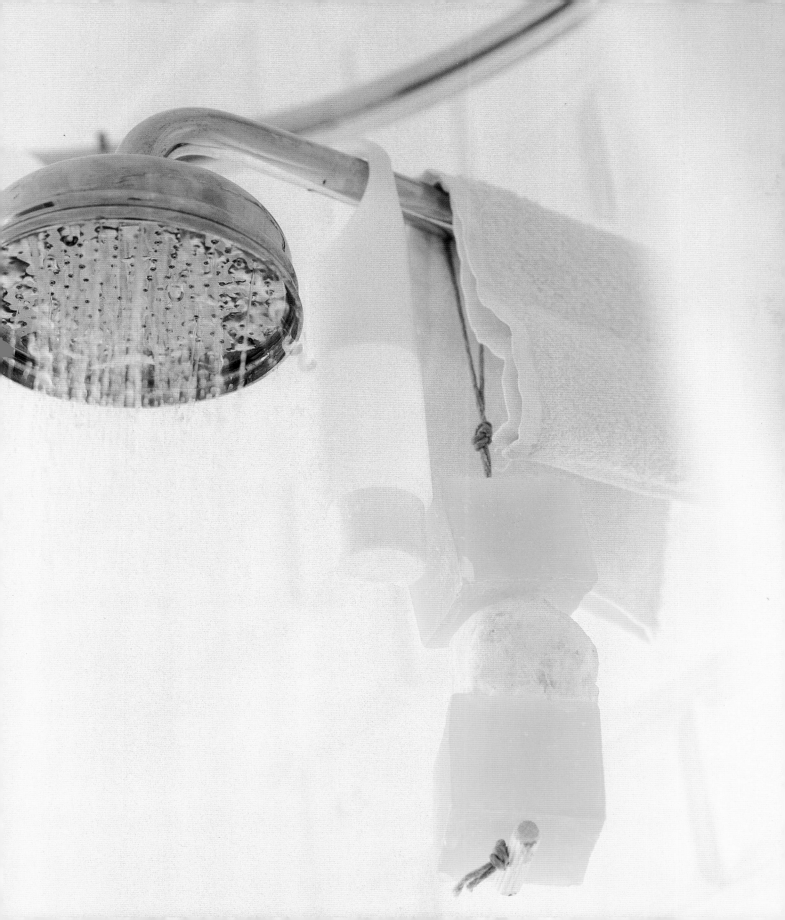

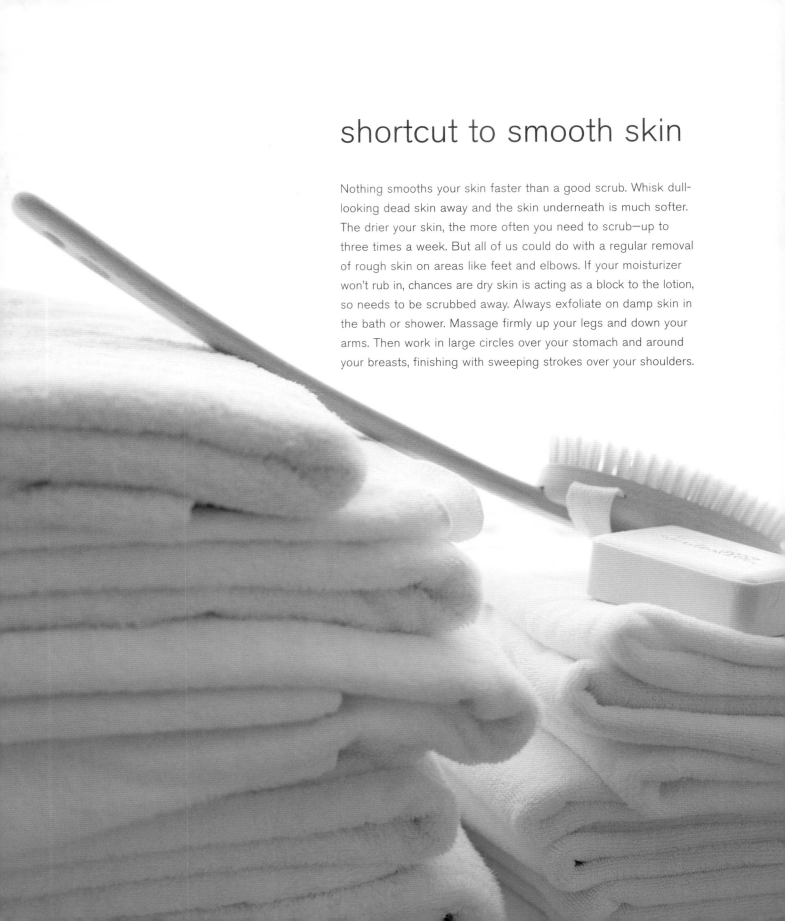

shortcut to smooth skin

Nothing smooths your skin faster than a good scrub. Whisk dull-looking dead skin away and the skin underneath is much softer. The drier your skin, the more often you need to scrub—up to three times a week. But all of us could do with a regular removal of rough skin on areas like feet and elbows. If your moisturizer won't rub in, chances are dry skin is acting as a block to the lotion, so needs to be scrubbed away. Always exfoliate on damp skin in the bath or shower. Massage firmly up your legs and down your arms. Then work in large circles over your stomach and around your breasts, finishing with sweeping strokes over your shoulders.

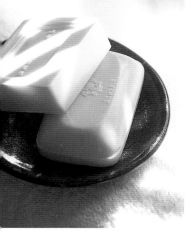

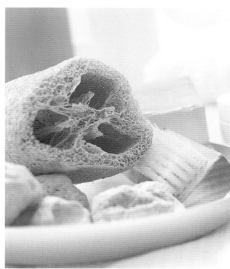

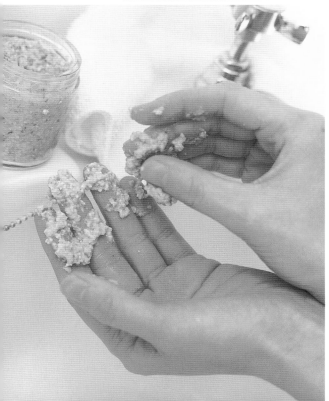

Pick the scrub option that suits the time you have.

ONE MINUTE

For the quickest option, choose an exfoliating soap bar to use in the bath or shower. But look for the word "gentle" as bodies don't like sharp, scratchy bits (no matter how natural they sound). Or press a handful of oats onto your usual bar of soap to make a no-cost alternative.

TWO MINUTES

Body puffs and exfoliating mitts are next in line. Body puffs are more gentle so suit sensitive skins, and also score marks for encouraging the weakest wash into a luxurious lather. Exfoliating mitts give a more intense scrub experience. They take seconds to slip on dry— and a few more to take off when wet. Just lather with your usual soap or gel and get to work.

FIVE MINUTES

For the softest, most luxurious scrub, treat yourself to a moisturizing mixture. These are usually either sugar or salt added to an oil base, which makes them very easy to do yourself at home. For a simple scrub, mix a handful of coarse sea salt with a teaspoon of any vegetable oil or runny honey, and massage onto damp skin before rinsing off thoroughly. Sensitive skin will prefer a handful of brown sugar mixed with oil or honey, as the effect is slightly less abrasive.

BATH OPTION

If you prefer to scrub in the bath, simply add a cup of sea salt to your water and scrub as you clean.

cellulite solutions that work

Pudgy thighs may be a common curse, but there's plenty you can do to improve the look of your lower half without spending a fortune on treatments.

I EAT AND DRINK YOURSELF SMOOTHER

The aim is to boost circulation and also strengthen the collagen fibers in your skin responsible for elasticity (meaning lumps and bumps are less noticeable below the surface). Fruit and vegetables will do just that as they're rich in antioxidants and vitamin C, so eat at least five portions a day. Dehydration is another reason circulation becomes sluggish, so drink two quarts of water a day to help flush out toxins.

2 BRUSH AWAY THOSE BUMPS

Without doubt, one of the best ways to improve the look of dimply thighs and bottom is by brushing your skin. The type of body brush you use is unimportant; it's the way you do it that counts. Sweeping strokes on dry skin in the direction of your heart will stimulate the skin and the lymph nodes underneath. Start on your legs, working up to your bottom, daily before your bath or shower.

3 KNEAD YOUR KNOBBLES (BUT NOT TOO HARD)

Massage will help break down and disperse the fatty cells below your skin's surface, and you don't need to spend a fortune on cellulite creams to get results. Make your own dimple-buster with one tablespoon of carrier oil (any vegetable oil from your kitchen cupboard will do), plus two drops of cypress essential oil (to stimulate) and two drops of juniper essential oil (a diuretic). Smooth on daily and then gently pinch and roll sections of your less-than-perfect flesh between fingers and thumb.

4 BURN OFF YOUR FAT

There's no escaping it. Any form of cardiovascular exercise will encourage your body to burn fat and tone up flabby muscles, plus it boosts circulation. For best results, choose activities that target your legs and bottom, such as cycling, fast walking, and running. Studies also show that bouncing on a mini-trampoline not only gives good cardio (without putting stress on your joints), but also helps boost your lymphatic system (the one responsible for getting rid of toxins). Do it daily for at least five minutes for best effects.

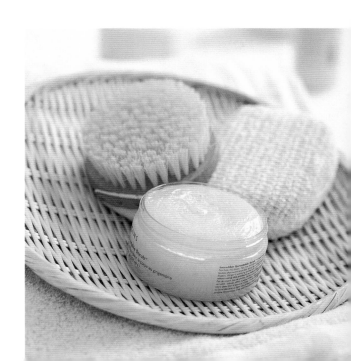

Sweeping strokes in the direction of your heart will stimulate the skin and the lymph nodes underneath.

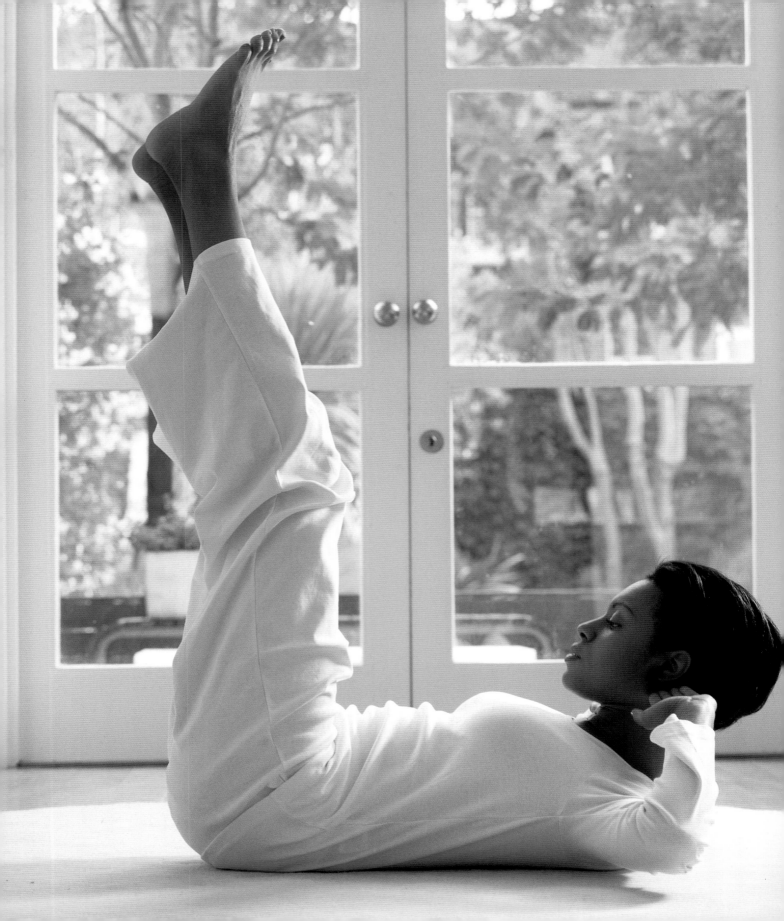

five ways to a flatter stomach

1 Avoid foods that cause bloating, such as beans, lentils, mushrooms, onions, wheat, and all carbonated drinks. You want to be eating plenty of easily digestible food such as plain bio yogurt, eggs, and oats, plus leafy salads rather than root vegetables. It's also a good idea to peel the skin off fruit, as it can be hard to digest, causing the dreaded gas. Talking of gas, high-fiber foods are also bad news for flat stomachs, so if you've got a tight dress to fit into, limit (or cut out) your high-fiber intake 24 hours before your big night.

2 Even if you eat the most easily digestible food, if you shovel it down, you'll still end up with a big belly. A major cause of bloating is eating too fast, or eating when you're stressed. And beware of talking non-stop at mealtimes as you'll be taking in gulps of air between mouthfuls that go straight to your stomach. So calm down, chew slowly, and concentrate on the food in front of you. And don't leave it too long between meals—the reason why most of us eat too fast is because we're so hungry.

3 Both pilates and yoga have a move that involves contracting your stomach so it remains drawn in during exercise. Easy to do any time, it's a great invisible stomach-muscle strengthener. Breathe in and pull up all the way from your pelvic floor muscles to your lower abdomen (imagine you're trying to stop yourself mid-flow on the toilet). The area above your navel should continue to move freely as you breathe. Hold this upward, inward contraction for 10–20 breaths—and repeat whenever you remember.

4 You may not have time for a hundred sit-ups a day as boasted by some six-pack-owning celebrities, but you actually get better results doing fewer high-quality crunches than lots of tired, out-of-breath ones. The trick is to target your stomach from different angles so you're using all your muscles, not just the same ones over and over again. To strengthen your entire stomach area, try the following.

□ Lie on the floor with your hands by your ears and legs straight up in the air. Tighten your abdominals, breathe out, and curl your shoulders off the floor, being careful not to pull on your neck. At the same time, bring your legs and pelvis toward your ribcage, using your lower abdominals to lift you (not the swing of your legs). Inhale, lower, and repeat ten times.

□ In the same position, tighten your abdominals, breathe out, and raise your right shoulder and elbow up toward the outside of your left thigh. At the same time, bend your left knee and bring your thigh toward your ribcage, again using your abdominals to do the work. Inhale, lower, and repeat on each side ten times.

5 If you suffer from bloating, pinpoint potential problem foods by keeping a record for a week of what you eat and how you feel 45–60 minutes afterward. Nutritionists believe that one in three of us may have a food intolerance, and simply by avoiding the problem you can reduce any bloating dramatically. Common bloat-causers include starchy foods such as potatoes, wheat, grains, and yeast. Alternatively, visit a nutritionist for a food intolerance test.

(easy) natural remedies for your body

□ The natural bleach in lemon will lighten red skin on your elbows and heels. Cut a lemon in half crosswise, squeeze out the juice, and rest your elbows or heels in each half for ten minutes.

□ Olive oil is contained in many prestige beauty products, so why not use it in its purest form straight from the bottle? Smooth on after a bath or shower and it will lock the moisture into your skin.

□ Add 4–5 drops of essential oil to a tablespoon of light olive oil (or any vegetable oil in your kitchen cupboard) to make a rich moisturizer with extra healing properties. Lavender is perfect for use before bedtime and also helps heal blemishes. Mandarin oil works well on stretch marks as it speeds up cell regeneration, and citrus oils such as grapefruit or lemon will wake you up in the morning.

□ Empty the contents of a vitamin E oil capsule and mix with a few drops of olive oil before massaging into your cuticles to encourage healthy new growth.

□ To soothe dry skin and eczema, put a handful of uncooked oatmeal in a large cotton handkerchief, hold all four corners together, and let your bath water run through it. The milky water it produces is a great softener and healer for sore and irritated skin.

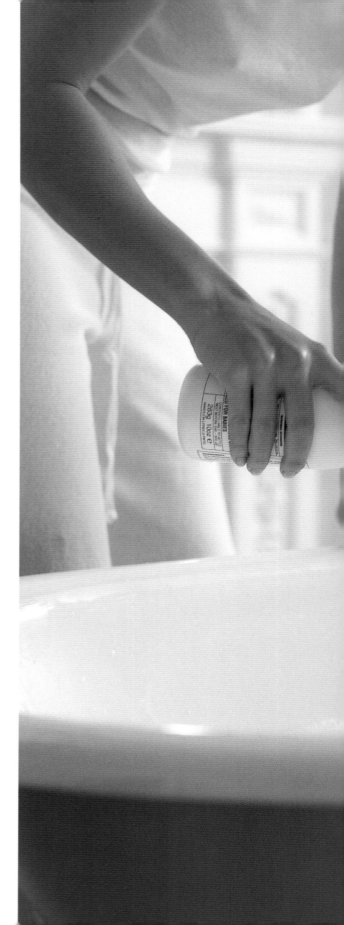

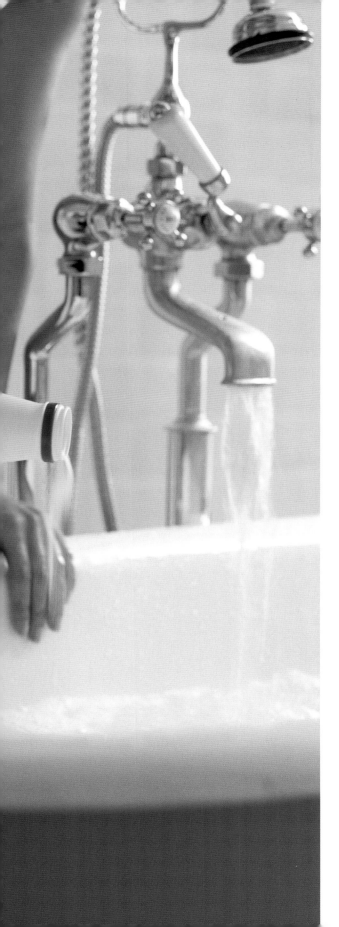

▢ Lie down with a cold compress to relieve headaches. Add a few drops of either peppermint (for tension headaches) or rosemary and eucalyptus (for blocked sinuses) to a bowl of cold water. Swirl a facecloth around in the water and loosely wring out. Lie down comfortably and place the cloth over your forehead for ten minutes, refreshing it in the water as it warms.

▢ A teaspoon of anti-inflammatory sesame oil will soothe tired, stressed muscles at the end of the day. Or add a teaspoon of clove oil (a natural astringent with mild anesthetic properties) to a teaspoon of sesame oil and massage into sore feet at the end of the day.

▢ As another pick-me-up for tired feet, add four drops of peppermint oil (stimulating) to two tablespoons of aloe vera gel (non-greasy, anti-inflammatory), and mix together with a fork before massaging into your feet.

▢ Spa body wrap treatments are popular for detoxifying the body, plus they tone and tighten skin, improving the look of cellulite. Do it yourself at home by adding a cup of sea salt to four cups of boiling water. Stir until dissolved and add two cups of cosmetic clay (available from health and natural food stores). Mix and let it cool for 10–15 minutes while you take a warm shower to open your pores. Then dip gauze strips (bandages will do) into the mixture one at a time and wrap firmly (but comfortably) around problem areas. Relax for an hour before removing and jumping in a lukewarm bath.

▢ Other natural bath additives to help skin conditions are a cup of wine vinegar to soothe dry skin, a cup of powdered skimmed milk to moisturize all skin types (very Cleopatra), and a cup of epsom salts to soothe sore muscles at the end of the day.

15-minute manicure

Who has time for weekly manicures? Luckily this one lasts for up two weeks. The secret? It's all in the way you apply your polish.

1 Most importantly, you need to get your nail shape right. It should reflect your cuticle shape, so if the base of your nails are square, you want your free edge to be, too. Getting an even result is hard to do on yourself, so check when you've finished by turning your hand around. With palm facing toward you, look to see if the free edges of your nails are straight. If they look uneven, finish shaping from this angle. And avoid filing down the sides—simply use one light stroke to clean up any snags and prevent splitting.

2 Before you work on the other hand, massage cuticle oil into the nails you're just filed.

3 Place both hands in warm water and soak them for five minutes.

4 Tap your nails on a towel to remove excess water and then, using an orange stick wrapped in cotton and dipped in oil, push back the cuticles on each hand.

5 Smooth on your favorite hand cream and then copy these reflexology massage movements.

□ Starting at your wrist, with your thumb underneath and four fingers on top, gently squeeze and release up to your elbow.

□ Using sideways movements in one direction only, stroke over the top of each hand.

□ Press all around each palm using the thumb of your opposite hand.

□ Interlock fingers and then press into the knuckles of each hand with the fingertips of your opposite hand (this improves flexibility).

□ Gently pull each finger using the thumb and first finger of your opposite hand.

6 Dip a facecloth in cold water and rub the nails clean until they squeak.

7 Apply base coat and then two coats of polish. Forget the old three-stroke rule. The more strokes you use to apply your polish, the longer-lasting the result. Take your brush out of the front of the bottle so the side loaded with polish is facing away from you and ready to paint. For the first coat, don't worry about streaks—just make a base. Start by spreading the bristles out at the cuticle (there should be a tiny gap between color and cuticle) and then run the brush up the nail in one clean sweep. On the second coat, keep stroking until all the air bubbles are out and the surface is perfectly flat.

8 The slower you paint on your color, the less likely it is to chip. For the same reason, don't attempt to dry your nails under the heat of a hairdryer; this dehydrates the polish, shrinking the edges and causing it to chip.

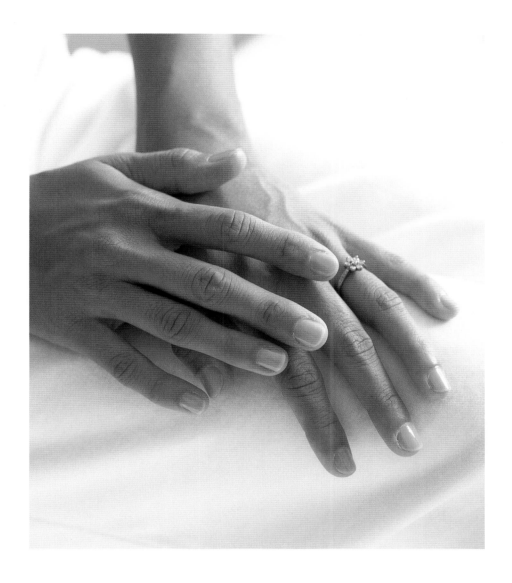

9 After ten minutes, smooth a drop of oil over each nail to protect your polish from knocks and dust while it dries completely.

IO Top coat wears off before base coat, so replace it every two days. Not only will your color look like new, your manicure will last twice as long, too.

Your nail shape should reflect your cuticle shape, so if the base of your nails are square, you want your free edge to be square, too.

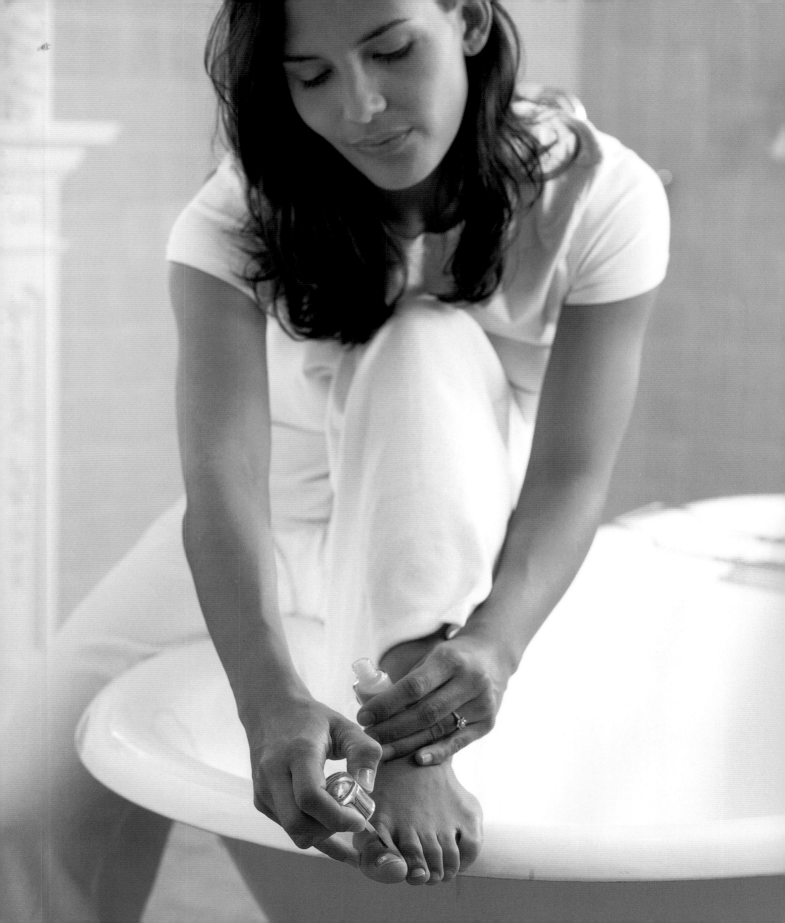

15-minute pedicure

Toenails come in for less grief than fingernails so you can expect
a pedicure to last longer. But up to two months? Now that is a luxury.

1 Place your feet in tepid water (hot water will make them swell) and add a squirt of liquid soap to cleanse. If your skin's dry, sprinkle in two tablespoons of baby-milk powder, which will loosen hard skin. Or add a few drops of eucalyptus essential oil to freshen up smelly feet.

2 Take out your left foot and, using a ceramic foot file (a pumice collects oil and loses its sharpness), get to work on hard skin. File across rather than up and down your foot so you don't risk removing good skin.

3 Trim toenails straight across with a nail cutter and then file to smooth the edges.

4 Massage oil into your cuticles and then use a body exfoliator (see pages 60–61 for do-it-yourself recipes) all over your foot to smooth away leftover dirt and dead skin cells.

5 Place your left foot back in the water and repeat on your right one.

6 Use a cotton-covered orange stick to push back cuticles and clean underneath the nails. Then buff the surface of your toenails to smooth ridges and remove any discoloring.

7 Massage in a cooling cream (don't use anything too slippery) and then blot away any excess.

8 To reduce swelling and wake up your feet for a night out, wipe an ice cube all over them until it melts.

9 Squeak the nails with a facecloth soaked in cold water in preparation for painting.

10 Twist a strip of toilet paper and weave it through your toes to separate them (far easier to walk in than foam toe dividers). Apply a base coat and then two coats of color. Follow the painting technique described for a manicure (see previous page) and remember to reapply your top coat every two days for the longest-lasting pedicure you've ever had. No time to wait for your polish to dry before putting on shoes? After ten minutes, smooth a drop of oil over each nail and then wrap plastic film around your feet to protect the color without smudging it.

NIGHTTIME NAIL TREAT

For a homemade heated hand and foot treatment, place a pair of cotton gloves and socks on a warm radiator. Before going to bed, massage a teaspoon of olive oil into your skin and then slip them on. The heat will encourage the oil to penetrate deeply as you sleep.

MAINTAIN YOUR MANICURE

Before doing anything dirty, run your nails over a bar of soap. When you've finished, wash your hands, and any dirt will come away with the impacted soap (and won't need digging out, which can damage nails).

21 instant rescue remedies

For when you're *looking* less than your best.

1 Woken up with flat hair and no time to wash? Simply hang your head upside down and rub your scalp all over using your fingertips (this is also great for headaches). Or mist with a little water, twist your hair into a high knot and secure with a clip or scrunchie. Wait an hour before shaking out and you'll have volume aplenty.

2 To beat morning frizz, again mist your hair with water and then smooth a tiny amount of serum between your palms (any more than a nickel-sized squirt is too much). Scrunch the curls back into your hair with your hands.

3 If you've woken up with a spot that's crying out to be squeezed (you can see the white sebum under the skin), then minimize damage for the rest of the day by opening your pores first. Either squeeze after a bath or shower, or hold a hot cloth over your face for five minutes. Wash your hands and wrap a tissue around the tips of your index fingers before squeezing gently. You want the spot to pop within seconds or the redness caused by your squeezing will look worse than the spot itself. Either way, dab on a little tea tree oil to guard against infection and then apply a concealer containing salicylic acid, an ingredient that's proven to clear blemishes and smooth skin.

4 An emergency tip for flaky lips. Press a piece of tape onto wet lips, gently remove, and the flakes will come away, too. Follow with a healthy dollop of lip balm to soften your lips.

5 Soothe redness due to heat or hormones by soaking a facecloth in ice-cold water, wringing out and placing over your face for five minutes.

6 To calm a red spot, place an ice cube over the top to cool the inflammation instantly. Another quick fix: dip a cotton swab in hot water and then neat tea tree oil before holding it over your spot for 30 seconds.

7 Celebrities use it, and so do makeup artists when they're making up a less-than-super model. A tiny amount of hemorrhoid cream applied onto the orbital bone below your eye will shrink under-eye bags instantly. But save this emergency measure for when you really need it.

8 Give dull skin instant energy by splashing with warm and then cold water. Repeat five times to boost circulation and bring color back to your cheeks.

9 Transform frizz into perfect ringlets by taking chunky sections, smoothing on a little molding mud or putty (the tacky-textured styling gunk that doesn't dry) and then twisting each section around your finger. And if you've only got five minutes just do the outer layer—it's the only bit everyone sees anyway.

10 When your hair needs a wash but you don't have time, just wash and blow-dry the front. Section off a triangle at the front and carefully lather and rinse before styling. This is the part that gets greasy faster, and what everyone notices about you first.

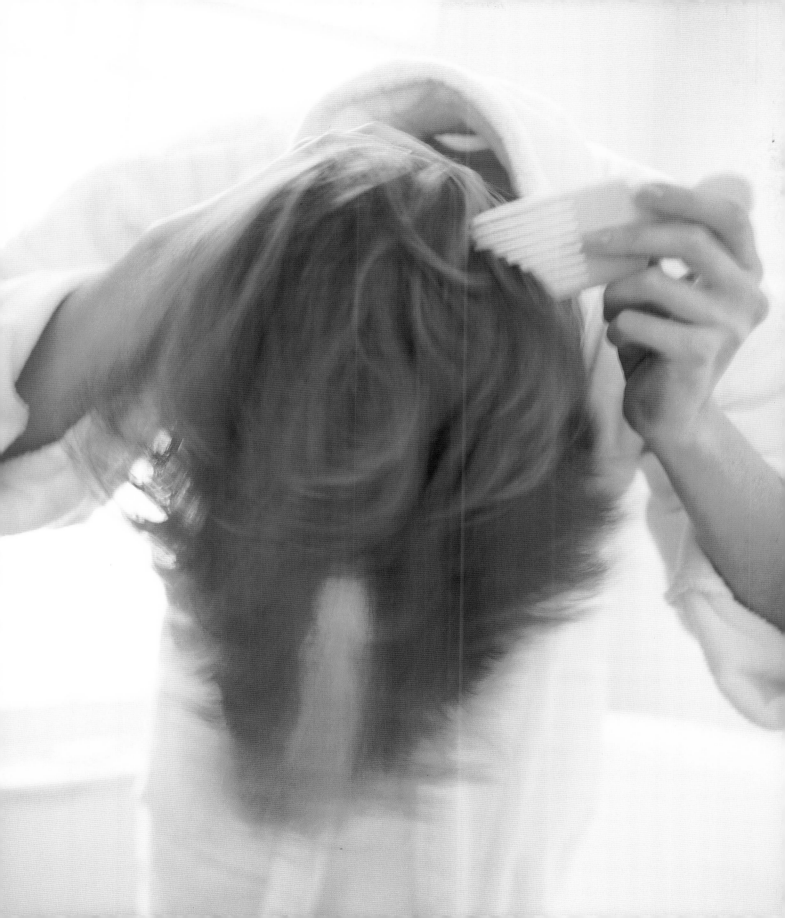

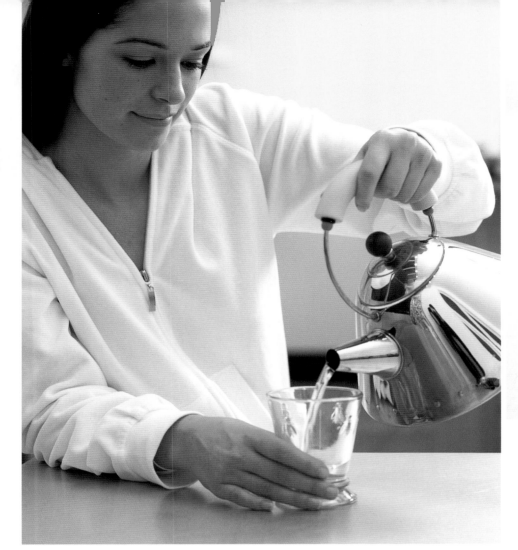

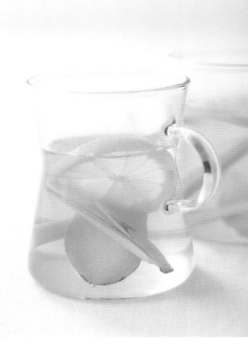

11 When last night's excess is still with you in the morning, start the day with a cup of hot water and a slice or squeeze of lemon to support your overworked liver. Follow with some deep breathing (see pages 106–107) to oxygenate your skin, and splash your face with cold water to wake up your mind and calm any redness. Ashtray hair can be sweetened by spraying some scent into the air and walking through the mist (shut your eyes). Drink a quart of water by lunchtime, and you should be feeling almost human.

12 Running late? A tinted moisturizer or concealer plus mascara and lip color is all you really need.

13 If you regularly wake in the morning with marks on your face, switch your cotton pillowcase for a satin or silk one. Dermatologists can actually tell which side of your face you sleep on by the lines left by your pillow, so minimize the damage by sleeping on something silky-smooth.

14 Woken up with flaking lips? Never try to apply lipstick over the top as it just accentuates the problem. Instead, try this makeup artist's trick. Use tweezers to peel away the loose flakes of skin gently and then apply a generous layer of lip balm. Leave to soak in before lining your lips and then filling in with lipstick.

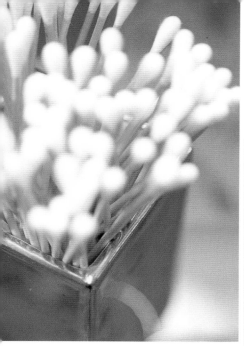
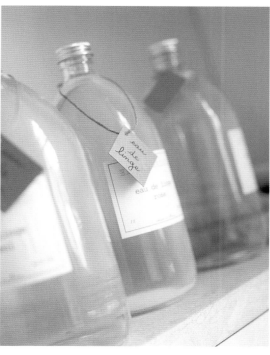
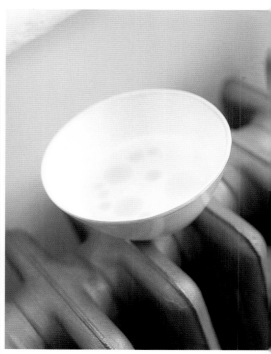

15 To banish a canker sore by the following day, apply neat peppermint, chamomile, or lavender essential oils with a cotton swab every 30 minutes (outside the mouth only).

16 Shrink under-eye bags with a spot of do-it-yourself lymph drainage massage. Lie down and, using the pads of your fingers, gently press under your eyes from your nose out to the sides of your face to remove excess fluid. Repeat five times.

17 No time for fuss? Ice-cold water splashed over your face is guaranteed to get your circulation going on a bad morning and bring a youthful blush to your cheeks (however, avoid this treatment if you suffer from broken veins).

18 Dry skin may be due to a moisture-sucking atmosphere. If you feel flaky, try putting bowls of water by all your radiators and surround yourself with well-watered, regularly misted plants.

19 If you have a shiny nose and forehead, invest in a T-zone control gel to wear alone or under makeup. These products contain powder particles that absorb oil to leave you shine-free all day. Or carry oil-absorbing blotting sheets, to dab on during the day.

20 To calm static and create shine, rub a fabric softening sheet over the surface of your hair.

21 If you have open pores, don't use moisturizer on your problem areas. They'll instantly look less obvious.

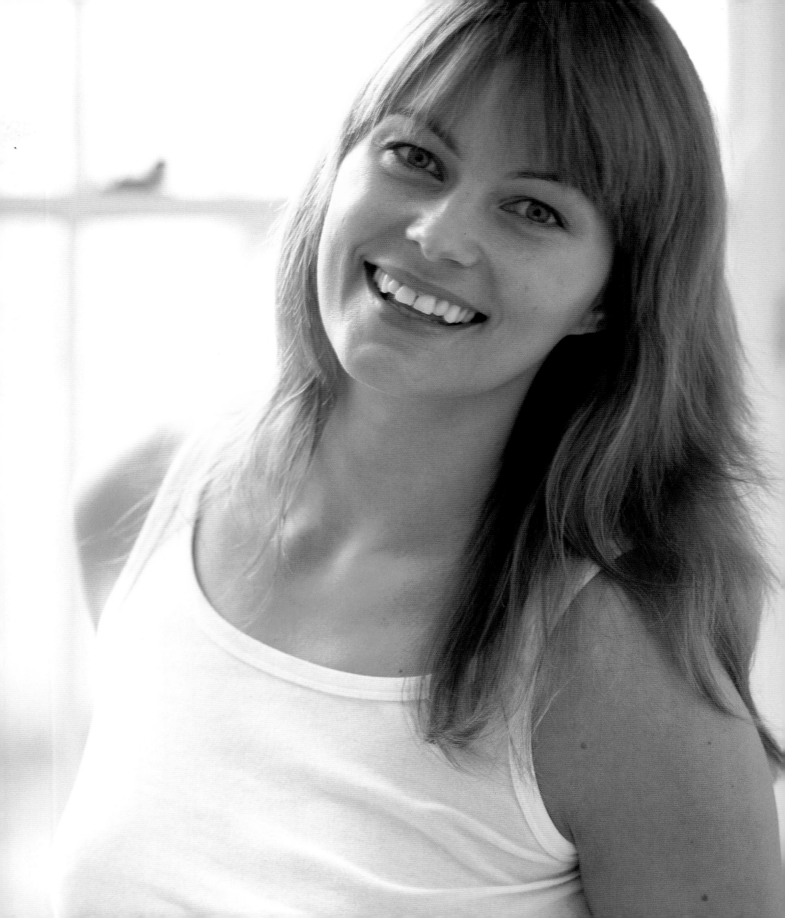

feel fabulous

healthy habits

A great way to feel in charge of a frantic life is to set up
what you want to happen each day. That means creating and
including activities that will improve the quality of your life.

The only rule is that these habits must be enjoyable,
so you'll want to do them no matter how hectic your
day. Make each one something you love, but which
you might normally forget to do because of all the
other chores that take up your time. The habits that
work best are ones that boost your well-being. That
might mean adding something new (like only eating
organic), or ditching something that you recognize
does nothing for you (like watching four hours of TV
a night). We all have habits we're not aware of that
cause us stress, and the more you can replace these
with healthy habits, the better your life will be. The
object is to look after yourself very well—extreme self-
care is the best habit of all.

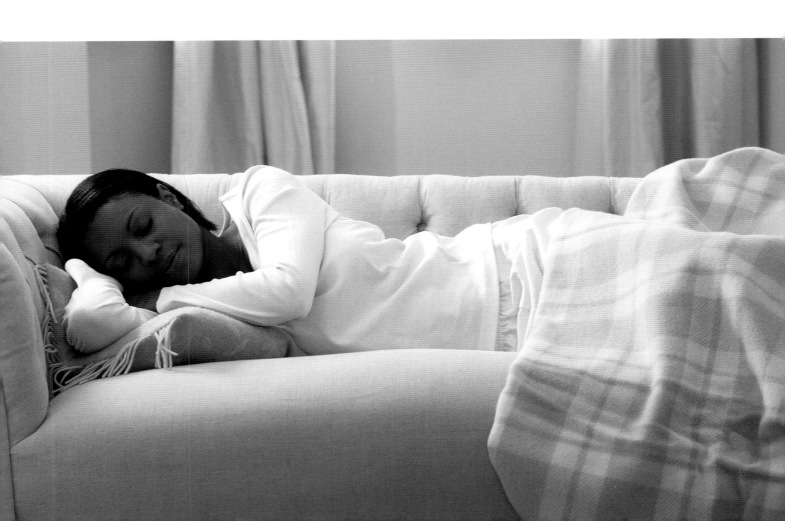

WHAT COULD YOU DO EVERY DAY THAT WOULD MAKE YOU FEEL GOOD?

The rules are simple. Make your habits

- □ simple and easy
- □ things that give you energy
- □ things you want to do (not think you should do).

And feel free to change them whenever you like. Remember: you're in charge of your own life, so it's up to you to make it enjoyable.

IDEAS FOR FEEL-GOOD HEALTHY HABITS

- □ Ten minutes of meditation, or simply sit quietly.
- □ Drink herbal tea instead of coffee.
- □ Do ten minutes of slow, deep breathing.
- □ Be in bed by 11 P.M.
- □ Use essential oils in some way.
- □ Take your vitamins.
- □ Indulge in a ten-minute self-massage.
- □ Limit your TV watching to an hour.
- □ Do ten minutes of yoga or stretching.
- □ Allow time to read things you really enjoy.
- □ Only eat foods that give you energy.
- □ Be kind to one person.
- □ Make yourself a fresh juice in the morning.
- □ Spend an hour playing with your children.
- □ Make a decision based on your intuition.
- □ Talk to a friend who makes you laugh.
- □ Play music you love.
- □ Have a hug or kiss.
- □ Go for a ten-minute walk in the park.

Now, over to you…

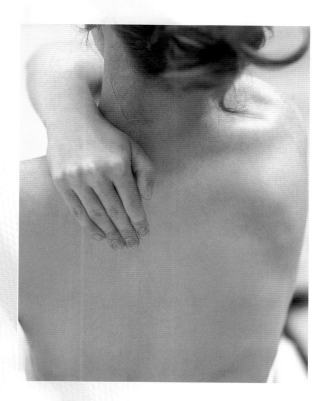

We all have habits we're not aware of that cause us stress, and the more you can replace these with healthy habits, the better your life will be.

why getting out is good for you

The benefits of nature are both physical and mental. Plants cleanse our air, taking the carbon dioxide we exhale and turning it into oxygen for us to inhale. No surprise then that plant-filled spaces are instantly relaxing and provide a peaceful escape from our otherwise high-tech day.

And the sheer size of nature can help put human problems in perspective. Many behavioral experts believe it's impossible to feel depressed when you're gazing up at the expanse of a bright blue sky.

GET OUTSIDE AND SPEND TIME WITH NATURE
Lie on your back in the park at lunchtime and watch the clouds. It won't matter how many people are around you, you'll feel instantly alone. Watching water is also very calming, so sit by a river or stream and

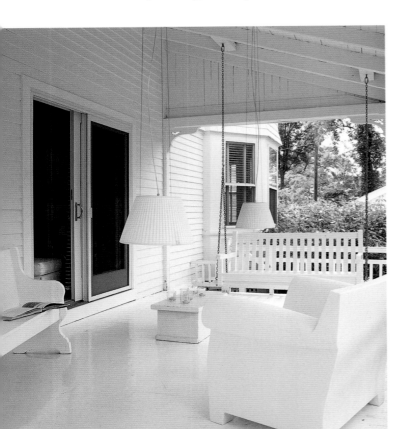

concentrate your mind on its movement. Nature can also benefit your well-being when you're indoors, so place plants around your home and in your office. Research has found they absorb common pollutants such as formaldehyde, and because plants pump out water, they'll also help counteract low humidity caused by air-conditioning and central heating.

THE SUN (IN MODERATION) IS GOOD FOR YOU
Vitamin D is formed on our skins by direct sunlight. A 15-minute walk in sunlight every day during summer is all you need to store enough vitamin D to take you through winter. Our immune systems rely on vitamin D to help prevent infections, plus it's necessary for calcium absorption in the gut. Calcium not only gives you healthy bones and teeth, but helps release the feel-good hormone serotonin, which boosts your mood and helps you sleep. It also has a calming effect on the nervous system, which is why we always feel positive after sun exposure. Although you can get your vitamin D fix in other ways (from foods such as fortified cereals, oily fish, egg yolk, cheese, and butter), the vitamin D your body makes from ultraviolet rays is the most effective. So, as many of us work and live in high-rise cities where sunlight is getting harder to find, counteract a lack of light by spending more time in open spaces (even on overcast days), and increase your consumption of vitamin D-rich foods as the days get darker.

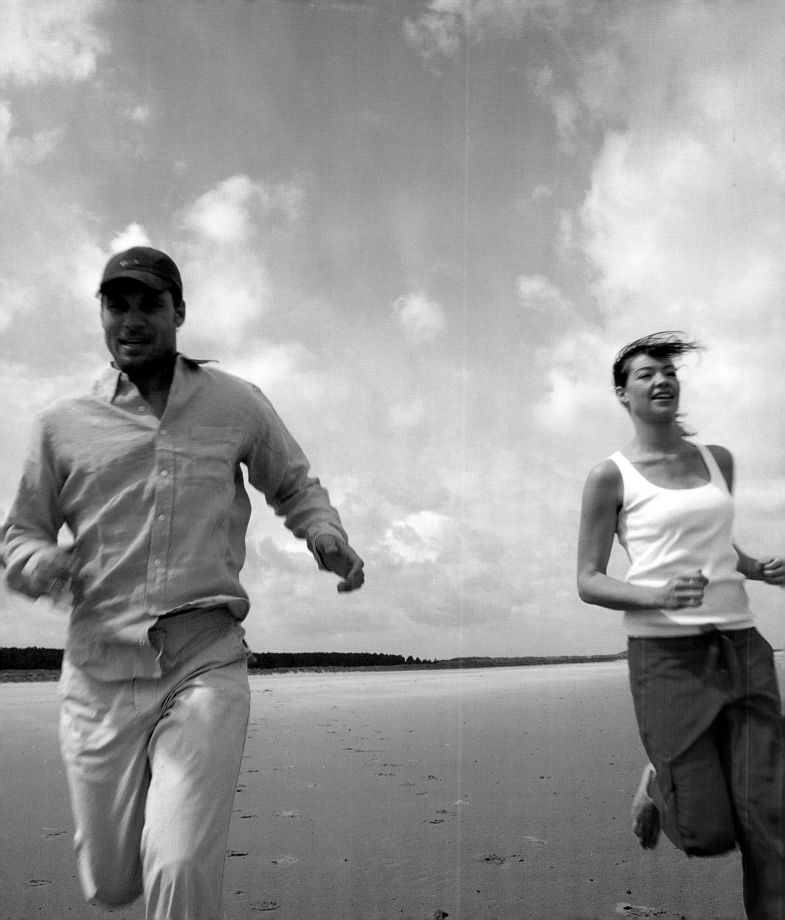

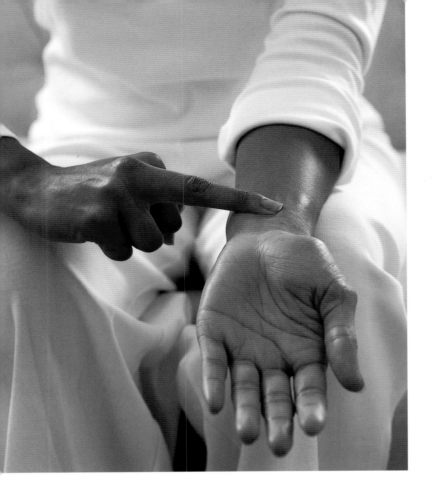

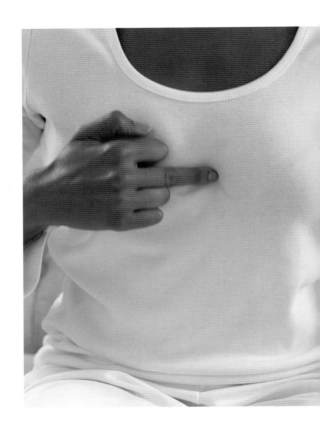

self-help acupressure

Acupressure, part of Chinese medicine, has been used for thousands of years to ease minor ailments. Like acupuncture, it works on the idea that health problems are caused by blockages of energy in the body. By releasing the block, energy can move freely again. But, while acupuncture uses fine needles, acupressure works by simple fingertip pressure. If you're pregnant, consult a qualified practitioner before treating yourself.

Do-it-yourself acupressure is easy to practice any time, anywhere. Simply apply steady, firm pressure, using the tip of your middle finger, to the acupressure point related to your problem. Hold your finger at a right angle to the surface of your skin (if you have long nails, you could use your knuckle instead). If

you're not sure you've hit the right spot, probe until you feel a sore sensation—the pressure should feel slightly uncomfortable. Hold each pressure for 20 seconds, release for 10, and then press for another 20 seconds. Repeat up to six times, plus a couple of times over the next few hours until your symptoms ease.

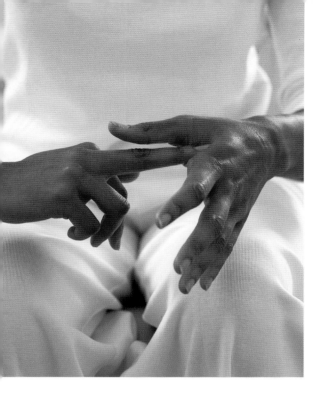

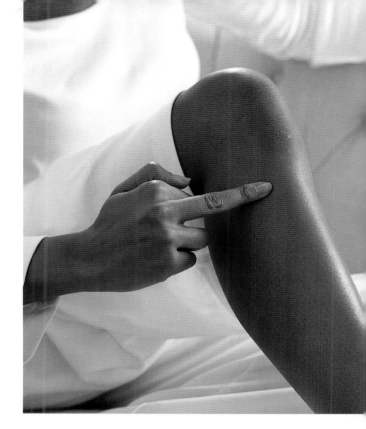

STRESS

Find the point between two tendons on your inner arm, about three finger widths from the wrist crease (see far left). Clench your fist so you can see the tendons, and relax it again before applying pressure with the middle finger of your opposite hand. Repeat both sides.

ENERGY BOOST

This point is at the tip of each finger either side of the nail. Take the top of your pinky finger between the index finger and thumb of the other hand and squeeze firmly. Hold for a few seconds. Repeat on each finger.

TEMPLE AND EYE HEADACHES

The pressure point is between the first and second toes. With your thumb and index finger (thumb on top), press gently into the webbing of your foot. Then gently squeeze the inside of the big toe just below the nail, but softly as this may feel sore.

ANXIETY

The anxiety point lies on the center of the breastbone three thumb widths up from the base of the bone (see center left). Apply firm pressure.

TENSION HEADACHES

The point lies on the top of your hand at the center of the fleshy part between your thumb and index finger (see center right). Repeat on both hands.

EXHAUSTION

To combat exhaustion, find the point four finger widths below your kneecap at the outside of your shinbone (see above right). Repeat on the other side.

TIRED EYES

This pressure point lies on top of your foot two finger widths from the joint between your big and second toes. Repeat on the other side.

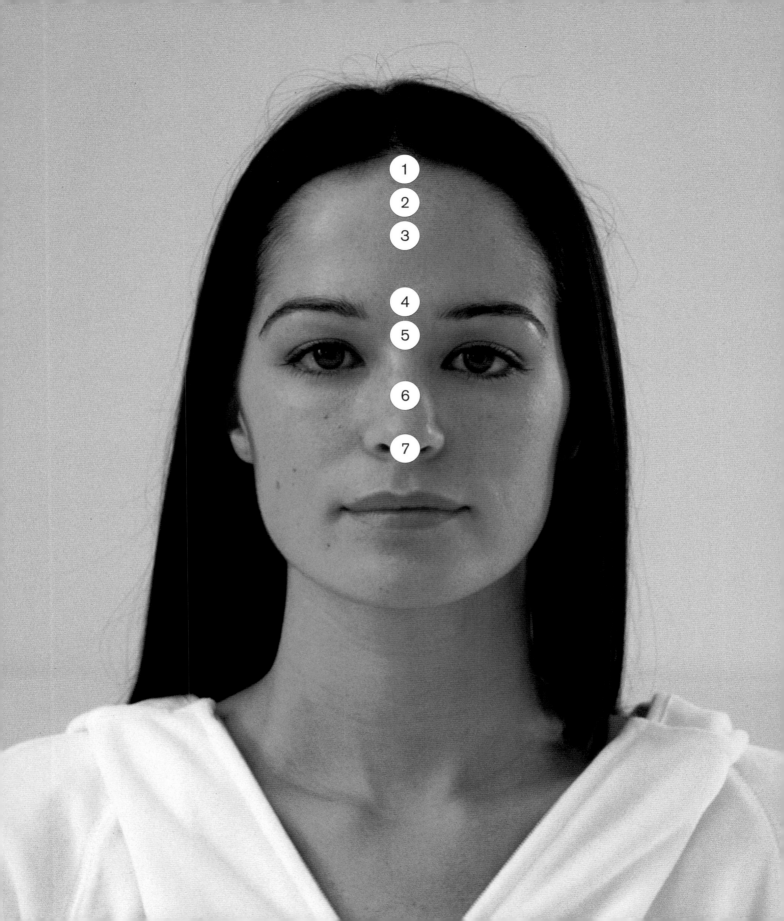

face reflexology

Face reflexology works more quickly and effectively than traditional foot reflexology because it activates your brain waves. A treatment stimulates the bloodstream and entire nervous system, while giving you a serious sense of relaxation. Using acupuncture points corresponding to nerve endings, it's also simple to do on yourself at home.

This sequence will relax and rebalance you after a busy day. There are seven points to massage. Apply medium pressure and work *very* slowly and rhythmically.

I Lie down for best results, or sit in a comfortable chair. Take a few deep breaths before you begin.

2 Starting on the first reflexology point just under your hairline (1), use your middle finger to circle around the point eight times. The movement needs to be calm and your working hand and shoulder relaxed. To divert your mind from busy thoughts, concentrate on an image of each point as you massage around it. Then circle in the opposite direction eight times.

3 Drop down one finger width and massage the second reflexology point (2) eight times in each direction. Remember to keep your shoulder and hand relaxed and the movements very slow.

4 Drop down one more finger width and massage the third point (3) eight times in each direction.

5 There's a small gap between the third and fourth points (4); drop down another finger width to find the fifth point (5). Massage eight times in each direction.

6 The sixth point (6) is at the soft part of your nose about halfway down, and the seventh (7) is on the tip of your nose. Massage eight times in each direction.

FACE MAPPING

Reflexologists believe that each part of your body relates to a corresponding area on your face. Putting pressure on these points is said to unblock the internal flow of energy within the related part of your body, releasing stress and toxins. Another way to make use of reflexology is to learn how to read your face so you can pick up slight imbalances in your body before they become a problem.

☐ Between your eyebrows relates to your liver. Too many nights out drinking alcohol can cause spots here.

☐ Problems such as broken veins on your nose can mean your cardiovascular system is under stress.

☐ Your cheeks are related to your lungs, and irritation or spots here are linked to too much diary in your diet.

☐ Around your chin is related to your reproductive system and hormones, the reason so many women suffer spots here during their period.

do-it-yourself body massage

Massage has been a part of healing for thousands of years (the oldest known massage book was written in 3000 B.C.). This is no surprise—massage encourages the release of endorphins that reduce pain and produce a feeling of calm, strengthens the immune system, improves breathing patterns, and boosts skin.

Before you begin the following sequence, take a few deep breaths, and as you do, cup both palms over your closed eyes. Relax your neck and shoulders and stay in this position for two minutes. (It's also perfect for taking a break during a stressful day.) Repeat each movement five times, and each time you apply pressure, breathe out. The key to self-massage is to work *very* slowly to relax your mind and body. Keep your eyes closed when possible and breathe deeply.

1 SCALP
Using the fingers of both hands, apply firm static pressure, making very slow circles. Spread your fingers wide and, rather than slide them over your skin, think of "moving" the scalp gently over your skull.

2 TEMPLES
With hands and wrists relaxed, press firmly into the soft part of your temples with your middle three fingers (where you will feel a pulse). Follow with little circles, keeping the movements slow and relaxed.

3 JAW
With your fingers around the back of your head, press your thumbs into the corners of your jaw. The right spot is around the middle of the ear in the soft part just under your cheekbones (if you move your jaw from side to side, you will feel the joint under your thumb). Relax your jaw and apply pressure into the muscle with your thumb, keeping the rest of your hands relaxed.

4 SHOULDERS
Use the middle finger of each hand to apply pressure into the sore spot of the opposite shoulder. Press very slowly as you breathe out and follow with small circles.

5 HAND
Make small, firm circles with your thumb in the center of your opposite palm. Then grasp one finger from the base, keep firm pressure, and pull straight out toward the fingertips. When you're about to slide off, squeeze the fingertip for five seconds before you release.

6 FEET
In a sitting position, hold one foot. Using both thumbs, "walk" along the center of the sole firmly and slowly.

7 LOWER BACK
In a standing position, using the fingers of both hands, massage any sore areas along the spine (don't come up too high or you'll put strain on your shoulders). Then hold flat hands on both sides of your spine and rub vigorously up and down to warm the whole area.

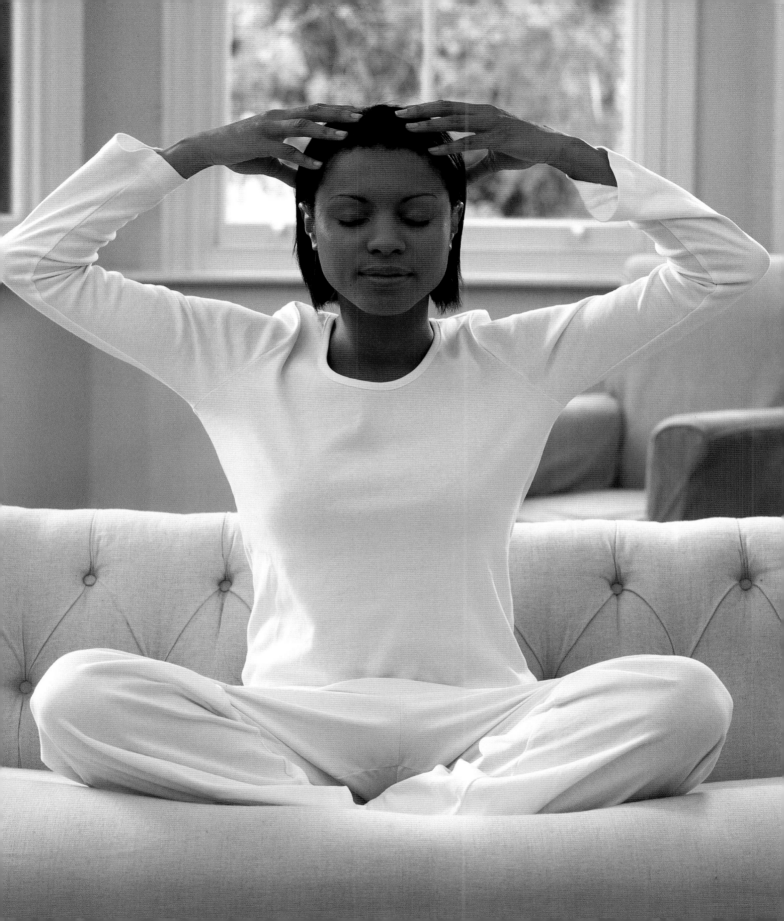

yoga moves for busy bodies

Most of us think of winding down as lying on the sofa watching TV, but deep relaxation is better achieved through gentle movement. That's because, as we stretch, our muscles release any tension that would otherwise stop us from feeling completely relaxed.

Yoga is the perfect wind-down exercise as it combines controlled breath (the body's natural tranquilizer) with movement, which calms your mind while energizing your body. The poses are designed to work every single muscle and joint, plus they also stimulate your digestive, nervous, and cardiovascular systems. The

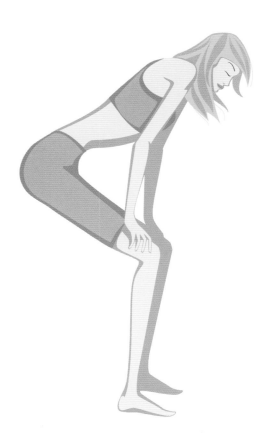

breath is deep and always through your nose. As a general rule, you inhale as you lift and exhale during downward movements. A feel-good addition is to smile gently as you inhale, as this not only allows the air to swirl around the back of your throat, but also works in the same way as the inner smile technique (see page 116). Most importantly, never hold your breath and keep it gentle—if you can't breathe freely, you're pushing yourself too far.

ALL YOU NEED

☐ An empty stomach—don't eat for at least one hour beforehand (wait two hours after a heavy meal).

☐ Comfortable clothing and bare feet.

IF YOU ONLY HAVE FIVE MINUTES IN THE MORNING

◀ STOMACH LIFT

This abdominal toner is the way yogis start their day and must be done on an empty stomach. Stand with your feet shoulder width apart and your knees slightly bent. With your hands resting on your thighs, inhale deeply and then drop your body forward as you exhale completely (until your lungs are empty of air). Holding your breath, come up to the starting position and pull up your stomach muscles as if you were trying to touch your spine with your navel. Hold for a count of three, release, and repeat.

CORPSE POSE

Begin and end any yoga sequence by lying flat on the floor with your arms a little away from your sides and your chin tucked slightly toward your chest to lengthen your neck. Imagine your spine relaxing into the floor, close your eyes, and focus on breathing in and out through your nose. This is a wonderful way to end your day as it allows your heartbeat to return to normal while circulating fresh air through your body.

IF YOU HAVE LONGER

OVERHEAD STRETCH

From the Corpse Pose, stretch your spine by bringing your arms above your head and interlocking your fingers. Inhale and stretch your arms toward the wall behind you. On the next inhalation, stretch your toes toward the opposite wall to stretch your whole body.

CHEST HUG

Ease a stiff back by bringing your knees toward your chest and holding on just below them. Inhale, and on the exhale bring your knees a little closer to your chest. Repeat five times.

▼ BACK LIFT

To soothe backache (and tone your bottom), bend your knees with feet flat on the floor, hip width apart and close to your body. Arms are by your sides with palms flat—your fingertips should almost touch your heels. Inhale, and on the exhale, lift your spine off the floor, tilting your pelvic bone and rolling up vertebra by vertebra. Keep your chin slightly tucked in and your shoulders on the floor so you feel your chest open. Take five gentle breaths and roll back the same way.

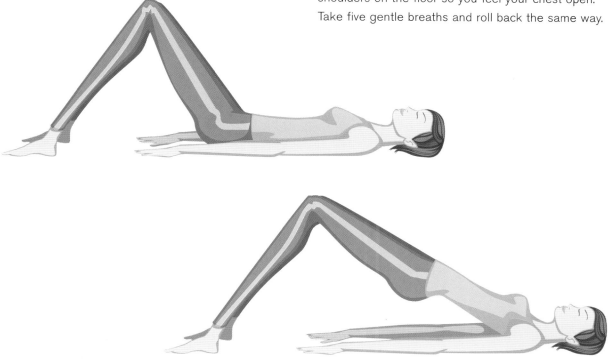

HAMSTRING STRETCH ▶

Improve flexibility in the back of your legs by coming up
to a sitting position with both legs straight out in front of you.
Inhale, lift your spine, and reach your hands straight up above
you. Exhale and bend forward from the hips (not the waist),
placing your hands as far down your legs as you can. Soften
your knees slightly, relax, and hold for five gentle breaths.

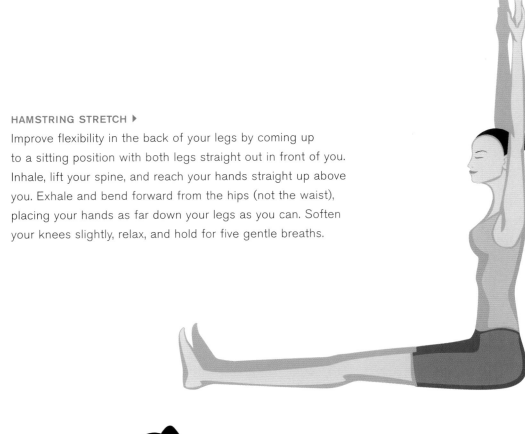

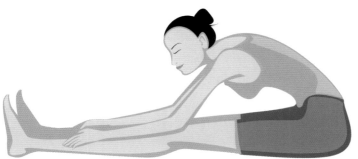

KNEE TWIST

To relieve tightness in the lower back, lie down with
your arms out to the sides and palms flat on the floor.
Inhale, and on the exhale take both knees over to the
right, keeping your shoulders on the floor and turning
your head to the left. Take five gentle breaths, come
up on an inhale, exhale and repeat on the other side.

THE CAT

Great for strengthening the spine and easing backache.
Start on all fours with hands below your shoulders
and knees below your hips. Inhale, and relax your back
down into its natural curve with your head lifted. Then
exhale, drop your head, and curl your back up. Repeat
five times, keeping the movements slow and gentle.

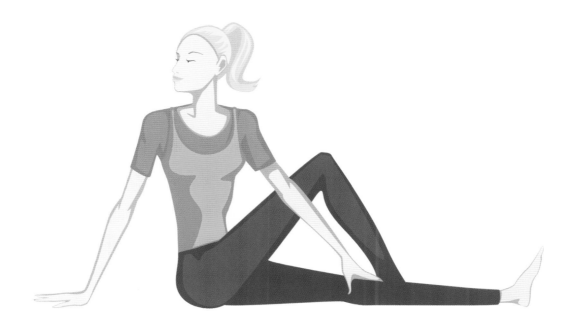

▲ SITTING TWIST

This pose will improve the flexibility in your back and spine while toning your waist. Begin as for the Hamstring Stretch, sitting tall with your legs out in front of you. Lift your right foot over your left thigh so that your foot is flat on the floor just above your knee and place your right hand behind your back. Inhale and lengthen your spine, bringing your left hand over the outside of your right knee. Exhale, and slowly turn your head over your right shoulder, twisting your entire upper body in the same direction. Continue to breathe gently five times and then slowly turn back and repeat the Sitting Twist on the other side.

HIP STRETCH

Perfect for anyone who spends their day sitting at a desk, this will ease tension in the hips and tone your buttocks. From a kneeling position, take your right leg forward, placing your foot directly under your knee. With your fingers resting on the floor to steady your balance, inhale, and on the exhale press forward and down gently until you feel a stretch in your left hip. Make sure your right knee is still directly over your ankle and hold the pose for five breaths before repeating on the other side.

AFTER STRETCHING

Finish by relaxing into Corpse Pose, staying there for at least five minutes (ten is better!).

Reminder: If you have any health problems or are pregnant, please consult your doctor before beginning any new exercise routine.

no time to exercise?

First, let's look at what you're missing. All exercise (whether it's serious boot camp aerobics or more gentle yoga stretching) will do the following.

- ☐ Increase your heartbeat.
- ☐ Give you more energy.
- ☐ Lower blood pressure.
- ☐ Ease back pain by strengthening stomach muscles.
- ☐ Release toxins and tension.
- ☐ Improve your memory.
- ☐ Lower your cholesterol.
- ☐ Tone and tighten muscles.
- ☐ Calm your mind.

- ☐ Improve your breathing.
- ☐ Strengthen your body.
- ☐ Help you sleep better.
- ☐ Improve your skin's condition.
- ☐ Make you look and feel younger.

And research shows that exercise also makes you live longer, so by exercising you're actually *making* time rather than wasting it.

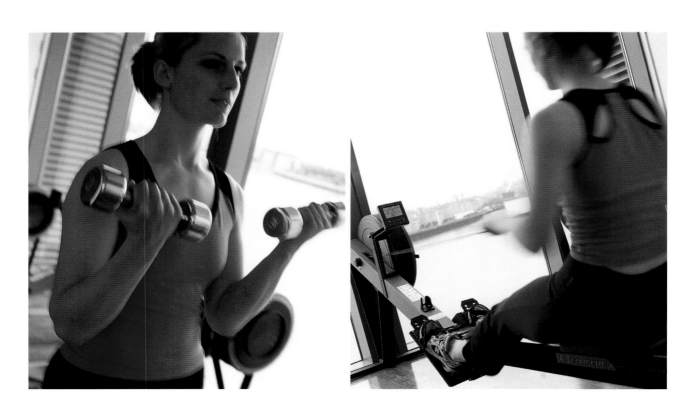

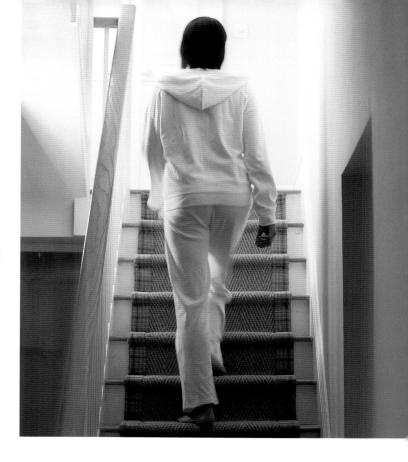

IF YOU HAVEN'T GOT TIME TO VISIT THE GYM, BRING THE GYM TO YOU

There's no need to invest in an expensive gym membership or home exercise equipment. Experts say it's not the twice-weekly run on a treadmill that brings the most benefits, but daily activity. A good recommendation is to walk 10,000 steps a day (about an hour and a quarter). This may sound a lot, but the little things add up: include using stairs instead of the elevator (approx 500 steps), 30 minutes of housework (1,500), and 30 minutes of lunchtime shopping (2,000) and you're almost halfway there.

Most importantly, include activities in your life that you enjoy and that also benefit your body—it's the only way you're going to want to keep on doing them. And while we're on the subject, sex burns on average 200 calories a session and also increases endorphins that make your hair, eyes, and skin shine. What more excuse do you need?

HOW TO MOVE MORE EVERY DAY

☐ Buy a basket for your bike and cycle to the shops.
☐ Park your car at the farthest corner of the lot, or three streets from work.
☐ Ditch the car and walk whenever you can.
☐ Take the stairs to the restroom three floors down.
☐ Put all your remote controls in a drawer so you have to move off the couch once in a while.
☐ Play with your children (or a friend's children).
☐ Never use the elevator, and walk up escalators.

☐ Take a ten-minute walk after lunch, and a 20-minute walk after dinner (weather permitting).
☐ Get off the bus or train one stop early and walk the remainder of the way.
☐ Walk your dog once more every day (or borrow your neighbors'—they'll be glad of the help).
☐ Give the office cafeteria a miss and walk to a deli ten minutes away.
☐ Get out in the garden at the weekend—weeding and pruning count as aerobic exercise.
☐ Go out dancing or take up salsa or swing.
☐ Volunteer to mow the lawn or wash the dishes (wearing dishwashing gloves, of course).

Include activities that you enjoy and that also benefit your body—it's the only way you're going to want to keep on doing them.

stretches for instant stress relief (without leaving your chair)

Tension in your body can be caused by both physical and mental stress. You may be sitting in the same position all day, or it may be your excessive workload that's sending your shoulders ear-ward. Keyboard users are also prone to soreness in the back, neck, and shoulders, not to mention eye strain.

These stiff-muscle-busters are the perfect 3:00 pick-me-up, but they'll also feel great any time you feel sore after sitting for long periods of time. The stretches marked with an asterisk (*) are particularly good for releasing the tight muscles that cause tension headaches. Do them all in sequence, or if you've only got a few minutes, choose the ones that target your area of tension.

CHEST STRETCH
Interlock your fingers behind your back, keeping your arms as straight as possible. Inhale, and as you exhale open your chest and pull back your shoulders. Hold for three breaths, relax, and repeat three times. (Do this standing up if your chair has a high back.)

NECK STRETCH*
Interlock your fingers behind your head with your elbows pointing out to the sides. Inhale, and as you exhale, drop your chin to your chest and bring your elbows together in front of your face. Hold for three breaths, lift up, and repeat three times.

▼ NECK SIDE STRETCH*
Inhale, and on the exhale slowly stretch your head down to one side, feeling a pull on the opposite side. Come up on the inhale. Repeat three times each side.

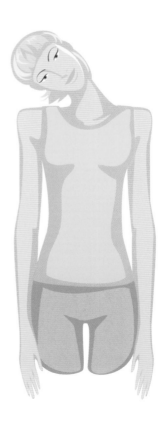

SHOULDER ROLLS

Place your hands on your shoulders with your elbows pointing straight out to the sides. Keeping your shoulders relaxed, breathe deeply as you move your elbows back and around in three large circles. Repeat in the opposite direction.

SHOULDER STRETCH

Interlock your fingers and stretch your arms up in the air over your head. Relax your shoulders, inhale, and then as you exhale look toward your hands and stretch. Hold each stretch for three breaths, release, and repeat three times.

UPPER BACK STRETCH

Interlock your fingers with your arms straight out in front of you and your head relaxed forward. Inhale, and as you exhale, push your arms out with palms facing away from you until you feel a stretch. Hold for three breaths, relax, and repeat three times.

▼ BACK STRETCH

Making sure you have room in front of you, inhale, and as you exhale, bend forward from the waist, relaxing your head down. Take hold of your ankles, inhale, and on the exhale gently arch your back to increase the stretch. Hold for five breaths before coming up.

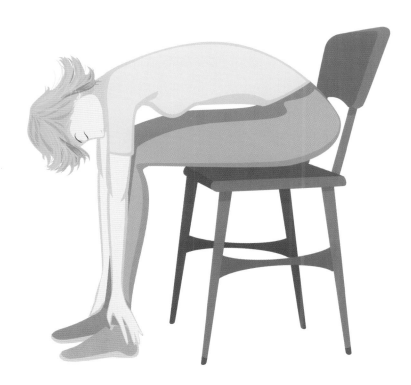

BACK TWIST

Sitting tall in your chair, slowly twist to the right from your hips so your chest faces to the side. Hold the back of the chair with your hand to help you stretch (but don't strain), and look over your right shoulder. Hold for three breaths and repeat on the other side.

▼ CALF STRETCH

Sit upright in your chair and lift your left leg straight out in front of you. Slowly flex and point your toe three times on each side.

FOREARM STRETCH

Lift and stretch your arms straight out to the sides. Slowly flex and extend your hands five times, feeling the pull on the upper and lower forearms as you go.

EYE STRETCH

Without moving your neck, look up to the ceiling. Now imagine you're watching a moving clock and follow the hand clockwise from twelve o'clock to one o'clock and then all the way around back to twelve. Repeat counterclockwise. Finish by rubbing your palms together to generate heat and cupping them over your closed eyes as you breathe deeply for five breaths.

FACE STRETCH*

You may want to do this when no one's watching! Inhale, and squeeze your face up tight, then as you exhale, open your eyes and mouth as wide as possible and stick out your tongue (try to reach your chin!). Now exhale with force, making an "ahh" sound. Repeat three times.

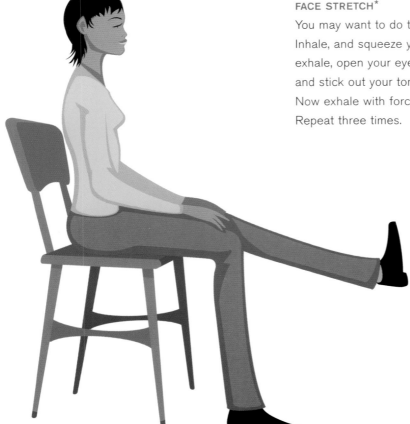

FULL ARM STRETCH

Take your right arm behind your back and bend it up, then take your left arm over your shoulder so your hands can clasp together behind your back (if you can't take hold of your hand, then try to touch your fingers). Breathe deeply as you hold the stretch for five breaths.

HIP STRETCH

Bend your right leg up in front of you and hold your knee with your right hand. Take your left hand and hold your right foot, keeping the ankle straight and in line with your lower leg. Straighten your spine to lift up through your waist and gently rock the right leg from side to side, feeling the stretch in your right hip (be very gentle, as this is an intense stretch). Hold for five deep breaths and repeat on the opposite side.

▼ FULL BODY STRETCH

Sit upright as before with your hands clasped loosely behind your back. Drop your head toward your chest so your back is rounded, and lift your left leg straight out in front of you. Inhale, flex your foot, and as you exhale, move your body gently forward to increase the stretch. Hold for five breaths, release, and repeat the sequence with the right leg.

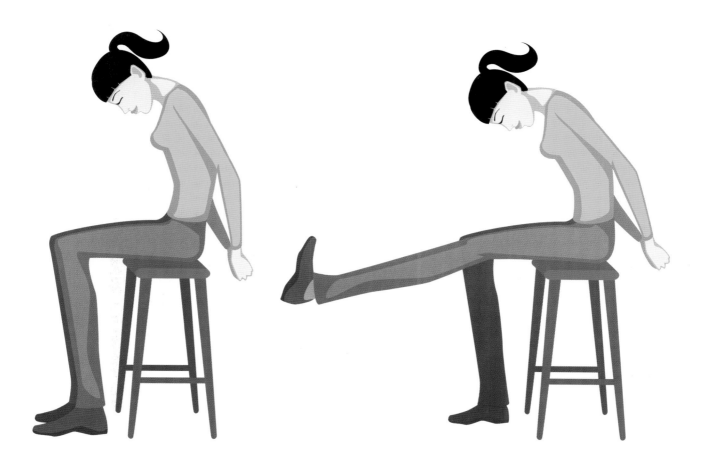

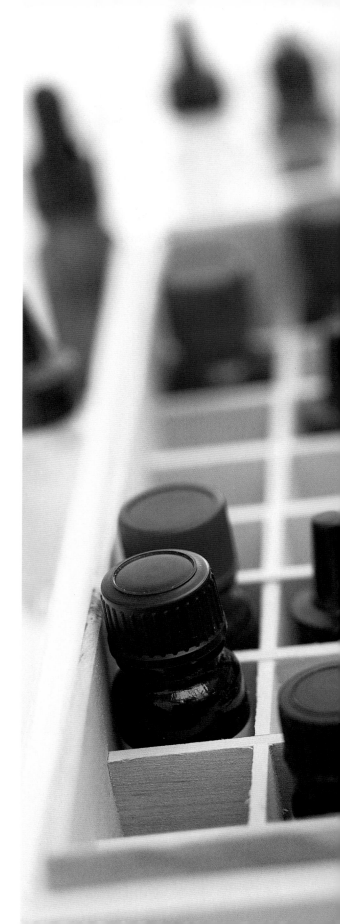

aromatherapy to help you through your day

Our noses work like a direct passage to the brain. The moment we smell a fragrance that reminds us of a positive memory, we experience the same good feelings again.

Natural scents go one better, as they affect the mind and body no matter what memories are associated with them. That makes essential oils some of the most powerful mood-altering substances available—and they're legal! Buy 100 percent pure oils and store in a cool, dry place.

WAYS TO SURROUND YOURSELF WITH SCENT

☐ Place ceramic ring diffusers above light bulbs in your home and office, or add a few drops of oil directly to the bulb. As it heats up, the aroma will be released.

☐ Invest in a small diffuser designed to slot into the lighter socket in your car.

☐ Sprinkle oils onto your linen, the corner of a carpet, or your pillow at night (there's actually no oil in essential oils, so they won't stain fabric).

☐ Add five drops to your bath water or shower floor, or sprinkle onto a wet washcloth and rub over your body.

☐ Burn scented candles or a diffuser in your office and home (clean diffusers with a little vodka between oils to neutralize any leftover aroma).

☐ Add a few drops of oil to the water compartment of your iron and the steam will scent your clothes.

☐ Make up massage blends (five drops to a tablespoon of vegetable oil) for a rich moisturizing treat.

☐ As essential oils come in tiny bottles, they're easy to use on the go. Sprinkle onto a handkerchief or simply sniff straight from the bottle.

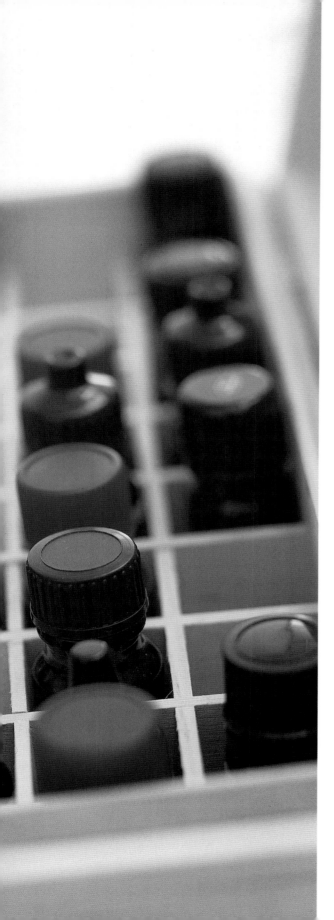

HERE'S WHAT WILL HIT THE SPOT

☐ Get going in the morning with orange, lemon, lime, or grapefruit essential oils, all guaranteed to clear the fuzz from the night before. For weekend mornings when you want to wake up gradually, lavender is perfect.

☐ If you're driving long-distance, using rosemary oil in a car diffuser will aid concentration and help you get to your destination safely, with less stress. Lavender will soothe road-rage nerves without sending you to sleep.

☐ Give yourself a wake-up call at work with cedarwood or peppermint. Again, if it's concentration you're lacking, rosemary will get you back on track. Sprinkle two drops on a handkerchief, lay it over the top of your computer, and the gentle heat will diffuse the oil into your space.

☐ Keep going at midday with a blast of peppermint oil to revive a tired mind. Peppermint is also good before an important meeting as it soothes and calms nerves. If you're suffering from low spirits, eucalyptus will lift you up, and stressed-out days will seem a little less frantic after smelling orange essential oil.

☐ Slow down at night by surrounding yourself with the scent of relaxing jasmine. If you're wanting to create a sensual atmosphere, sandalwood and ylang ylang are renowned aphrodisiacs and also smell very romantic.

☐ Prepare yourself for bed by adding chamomile or lavender oil to your bath water—perfect for tired bodies and minds. Sprinkle lavender on your pillow to insure a good night's sleep (it stimulates the part of your brain responsible for regulating sleep patterns), but use sparingly, as a too-strong aroma will have the opposite effect. If you've got a cold choose eucalyptus instead: it will aid your breathing in the night.

chill-out techniques

Too busy to breathe? Take a few minutes out of your
busy schedule to practice one of these relaxation tricks.

IF YOU'VE GOT TWO MINUTES

A big stretch will loosen up tense muscles, and
lengthening your spine not only feels fantastic, it also
creates space, enabling you to breathe more deeply.
Lie on your back with your arms stretched out over
your head. Interlock your fingers, point your toes,
take a big breath in, and stretch your arms and legs
away from you. Hold for a few seconds, relax, and
repeat three times.

Singing and humming relieve stress as they cause
relaxing vibrations in your throat. Hum to yourself
when you start to feel stressed, and after a busy day,
turn up your car radio and sing all the way home.

IF YOU'VE GOT FIVE MINUTES

You don't need to be in a calming environment to
meditate effectively. Simply zone out by watching
something repetitive like washing in a machine or
traffic from a bus window. Just soften your focus
and detach your thoughts for a while—you may be
surprised where they go when you let them wander.

Shiatsu massage works on your body's meridians
to influence the energy flowing through you. To find
your stress-relief point, slide your thumb between the
bones leading away from your middle and ring fingers
until you reach the center of your palm. Breathe in and
press your thumb into this point as you slowly breathe
out (if you've hit the right spot, you'll feel a dull ache).
For best results, press and hold six times on each hand.

Yogis relax into child's pose, as it calms and tones
the nervous system while gently stretching the neck,
shoulders, and spine. Kneel on the floor with your
arms by your sides, and bend forward until your
forehead is gently resting on the floor and your hands
are resting by your feet. Inhale and exhale as you feel
your breath slow and your body completely relax. Bliss.

The next time you feel stressed, laugh. Laughter
releases endorphins into your brain (the ones you
usually have to exercise to get), which reduce levels
of the stress hormone cortisol, relax tense muscles,
and boost your immune system. The average adult
laughs only 17 times a day (compared to 300 times
as a child), so do what it takes to lighten up. Phone
a witty friend, recall a funny memory, or share a joke.

IF YOU CAN SPARE TEN MINUTES

Progressive muscle relaxation is the most thorough
way to relax your body. Lie on the floor and, starting
with each foot, clench your toes tight for five seconds
before letting your foot go floppy. Next lift each leg
off the floor and hold for five seconds before gently
dropping it down. Repeat the tensing and relaxing
process all the way up your body, concentrating on
different muscles every time. Clench your bottom hard
and release, make a fist, lift each arm off the floor in
turn, and tense your shoulders up to your ears. When
you reach your face, close your eyes tightly, then open
your mouth wide, stick out your tongue, and make
a loud "ahh" sound. Spend at least five minutes in this

super-relaxed state, feeling the full weight of your body heavy on the floor.

With new technology providing ever-increasing ways to communicate, most of us are reaching attention overload, which is why it's important to do absolutely nothing once in a while. Go to any comfortable, quiet spot: your couch, your car, or a café, and simply watch your mind do its thing. Don't judge what comes up, just be aware of all the activity. Detaching yourself in this way frees your mind from the fear that stops you from seeing things clearly—this is the reason why solutions to previously unsolvable problems can come up when you least expect them.

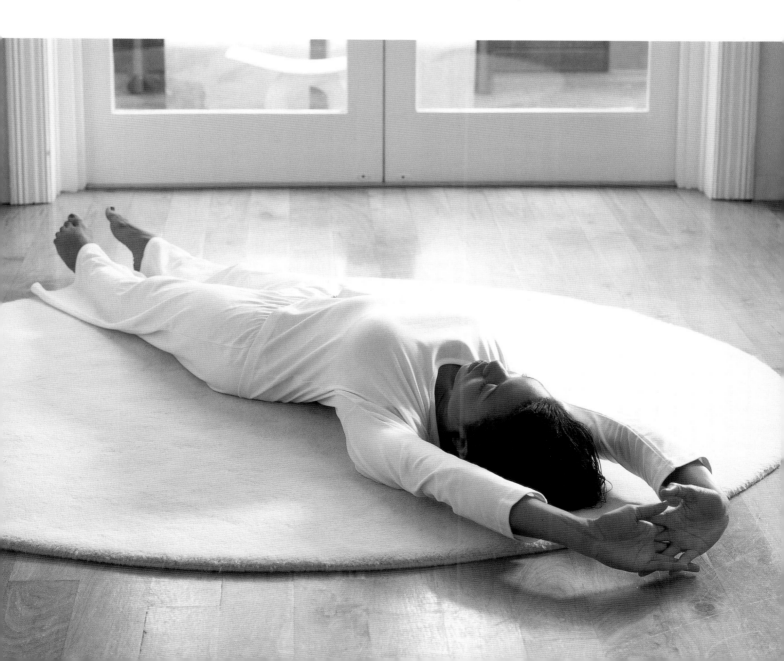

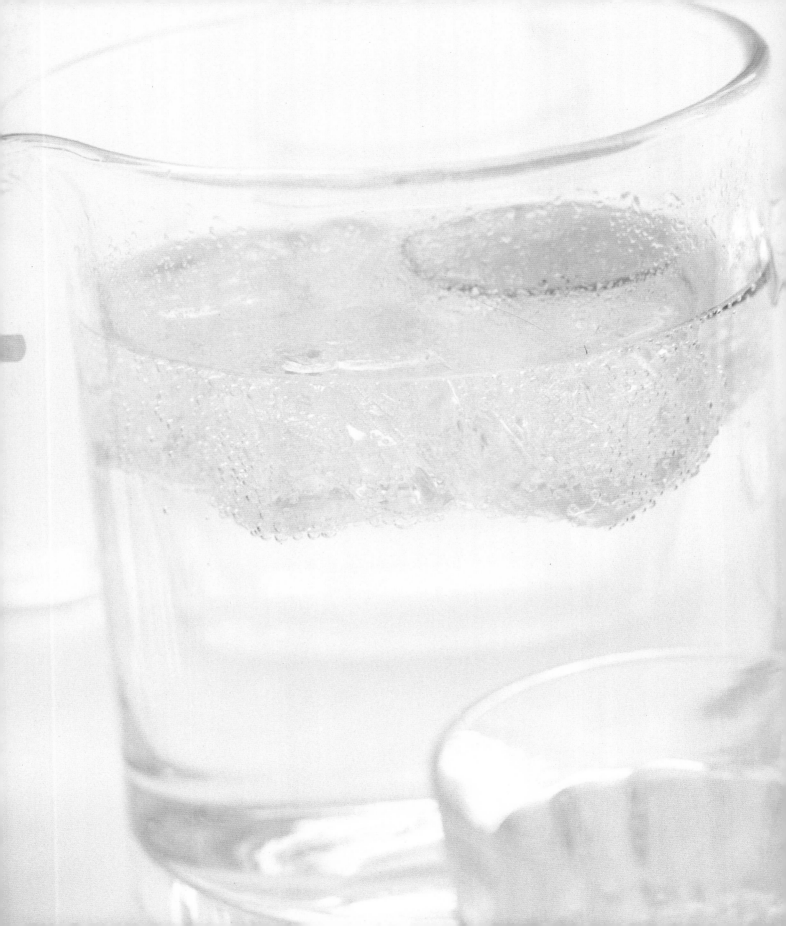

detox without trying

You don't need to live on lettuce leaves to feel the
benefits of a spa detox. Read on for the real-life way.

**DITCH THE LATTE AND START YOUR DAY WITH A GLASS
OF HOT WATER AND LEMON**
Just a few squeezes of lemon in a cup of hot water
will have a cleansing effect on your liver, unlike coffee,
which puts extra stress on your body by encouraging
your adrenal glands to work harder. The result is an
increased heart rate and slower digestion, neither
of which encourage a mellow start to the day.

EAT ORGANIC FRUIT AND VEGETABLES
The best way to reduce exposure to toxic substances
is to buy organic. Not only does organic farming keep
the air and soil clean, but fruit and vegetables not
treated with pesticides are also much more nutritious.
They may be more expensive, but absorbing all those
extra nutrients is so much better for your health.
If you can't buy organic, take the outer layer off by
peeling or scraping, so you know you've at least got
rid of surface chemicals.

DON'T IGNORE WHAT YOU PUT ON YOUR SKIN
Up to 60 percent of any substance applied to your
skin is absorbed, so if you're eating organic it makes
perfect sense to buy organic skincare and makeup,
too. You may experience an initial skin breakout, but
this is just your skin's way of cleansing itself of
chemicals, so give it time to adjust. Look for brands
that contain plant-based ingredients and organic
essential oils, plus natural preservatives (if any). For
guaranteed good-for-you beauty products, look for
certified organic products.

**DRINK YOUR WATER FROM A GLASS, NOT AN OLD
PLASTIC BOTTLE**
Once a bottle is opened, bacteria enter the top, and by
refilling it you're letting the bacteria multiply. And don't
leave a half-empty bottle on your desk without a lid,
as bacteria are attracted to the oxygen in the water.

LET PLANTS (NOT YOU) ABSORB COMPUTER RADIATION
Computers emit energy-sapping electromagnetic
radiation, so no wonder sitting in front of one all day
can leave you feeling drained. Luckily, studies have
shown that placing a plant by your screen can actually
reduce tiredness as the plant, rather than you, absorbs
the electromagnetic excess.

SWITCH TO ORGANIC DAIRY AND MEAT PRODUCTS, TOO
The average farm animal is fed growth enhancers
plus food supplements of animal origin, which contain
a high level of pollutants. Organic meat and dairy
products come from livestock fed their natural diet,
which means a far lower level of chemicals.

BEWARE OF CHEMICALS WHILE COOKING
You may think an alfresco barbecue is healthy, but
that burned kabob could contain potentially harmful
oxidants. Also beware burning your food in non-stick
pans, as they emit chemicals known as PFCs when
overheated. And if you use a microwave, let your food
stand for a few minutes before you eat it, as the
energy created during microwave cooking can affect
your blood and immune systems.

easy ways to eat better

Gone are the days when spa food meant spartan. What you will find at spas are plenty of the following, plus "mindful" eating: attending to your meal rather than eating in front of the TV.

START A NEW HABIT OF ALWAYS EATING AT THE TABLE
Light a candle and play soothing music to make it a feel-good ritual. Eat slowly and chew well so you really notice how your meal tastes. And wait ten minutes before helping yourself to another portion—your stomach needs this long to register how full it feels.

EAT FOODS AS CLOSE TO THEIR NATURAL STATE AS POSSIBLE FOR THE MOST HEALTHFUL DIET
That means plenty of whole grains (rather than their processed white equivalents), plus fresh fruit and vegetables. What needs to go, or be limited, are convenience foods such as ready meals, fast food, chips, cakes, and cookies. Give your body a spa-type break by going on a mini detox for the weekend. This not only makes you feel lighter and more energized, it also improves the condition of your skin and hair. Cut out meat, dairy products, convenience foods, wheat, salt, sugar, caffeinated drinks, and alcohol for two days. Beware side effects like headaches and sugar cravings as your body eliminates toxins. (The worse you feel, the more you probably need it.)

DRINK FRESH FRUIT AND VEGETABLE JUICES
It's a quick way to pack extra vitamins and minerals into your diet, and can count as one of your daily portions of fruit and vegetables. For best results and flavour, make your own at home using a blender or electric juicer. There's no magic formula here. Just combine your favorite fruit and vegetables and see what works best—soft vegetables like tomatoes and cucumber are the easiest to juice. Wash all produce first and drink immediately, as freshly squeezed juice doesn't keep for long (proof that making your own is so much better for you than the purchased variety).

USE HEALTH-PROMOTING HERBS, OILS, AND SPICES TO LIVEN UP YOUR MEALS
Try not to rely on salt and sugar (the secret behind those tasty TV dinners) to flavor your food. Add garlic to stir-fries for its immunity-boosting properties; it's antibacterial and antiviral, so helps fight off infection. Fry with sesame oil, which contains essential fatty acids to keep your heart healthy. And add finely chopped chili pepper to your food to aid digestion, help fight colds, and warm your body on a cold night.

STIR-FRY OR STEAM YOUR FOOD IN A WOK
This will retain most of its nutrients. The large surface area of the base allows heat to spread quickly, which means food cooks quickly without losing important goodness, or taste. Both couldn't be easier. To stir-fry, cut food into bite-sized pieces and use just enough oil to coat the inside of the wok—never use butter. Steaming is even healthier as it involves no extra fat and preserves most of the water-soluble vitamins that boiling takes away. Invest in some bamboo steamers to place above the simmering water. Don't pack your food too tightly or the steam won't be able to circulate evenly, and replace water with freshly boiled.

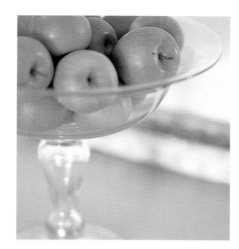

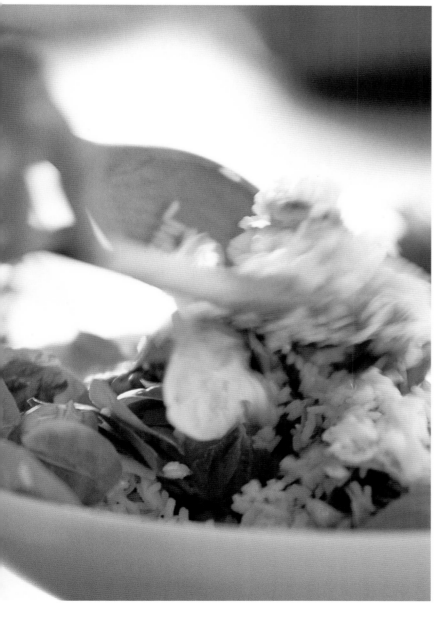

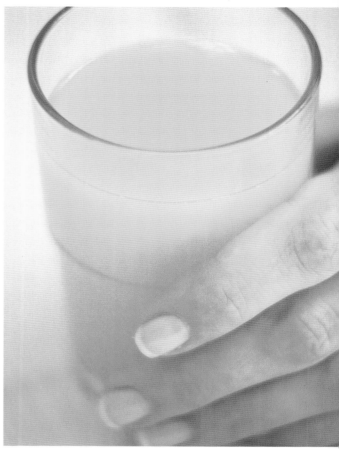

Juices are a quick way
to pack extra vitamins and
minerals into your diet,
and can count as one of
your daily portions of
fruit and vegetables.

just a perfect day

Looking after yourself—all day—not only makes you feel great, it also boosts your self-esteem, because you're treating yourself like someone who's *worth* looking after.

RISE AND SHINE

Take a few minutes to think positively about the day ahead. The minute your eyes open, ask yourself: What is today's exciting thing? Having at least one thing to look forward to sets an optimistic tone for the rest of the day. If life seems aimless, ask yourself: For what or whom am I getting up today? Take control of your life by deciding where to place your attention that day.

Still in bed, practice some energizing deep breaths. Most of the time we breathe shallowly, but breathing more deeply brings a rich supply of oxygen to the blood. This energizes your body, leaving you more clear-headed for the day ahead. Imagine your lungs are divided into three sections: lower, middle, and upper. One complete breath in fills each section with air; one complete breath out leaves you feeling empty.

I With hands resting on your abdomen, feel it rise as you inhale deeply through your nose, drawing air into the lower part of your lungs.

2 Move your hands to rest just below your ribs, and without pausing continue your inhalation, feeling a smaller rise under your hands.

3 Cross your arms and place your fingers just below your collarbone as you continue your inhalation, drawing air into the upper part of your lungs. Again, your collarbones should rise slightly.

4 Pause for a few seconds and then exhale slowly from the upper, middle, and lower part of your lungs, until you feel completely empty of air. Repeat five times with your arms resting by your sides.

You may have to wake up 30 minutes earlier than normal, but making time for the things you enjoy can change the entire course of your day. What start to the day usually means you have a good one?

☐ Playing your favorite CD while dressing?
☐ Sprinkling essential oils in the shower?
☐ Eating an energy-packed breakfast?
☐ Taking a walk or going for a swim?
☐ Wearing your best underwear?

Even simple changes such as waking up to a relaxing CD rather than a nerve-jarring alarm can make all the difference to your morning.

LUNCHTIME LAW

Whatever your workload, always eat lunch away from your desk. If your body's eating and your mind's working, you're completely out of balance. Plus you won't even notice what you've put in your mouth—a waste of a good meal. After lunch, take a ten-minute walk outside to encourage your body to digest the food you've just eaten. Studies show that gentle exercise after eating burns up serious calories, plus the fresh air will clear your mind for the afternoon.

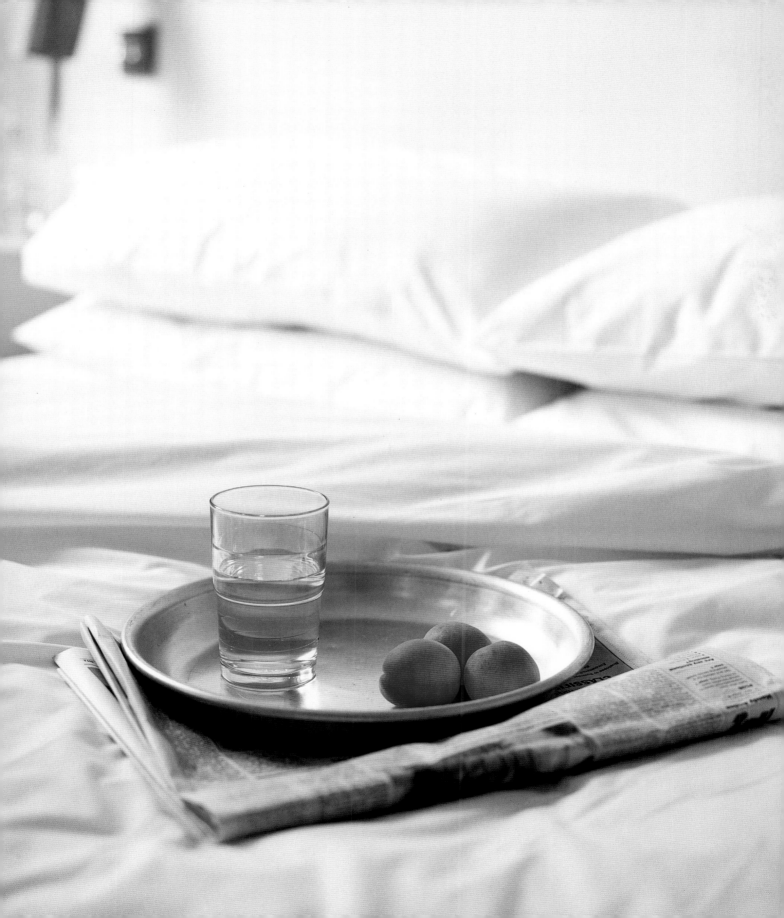

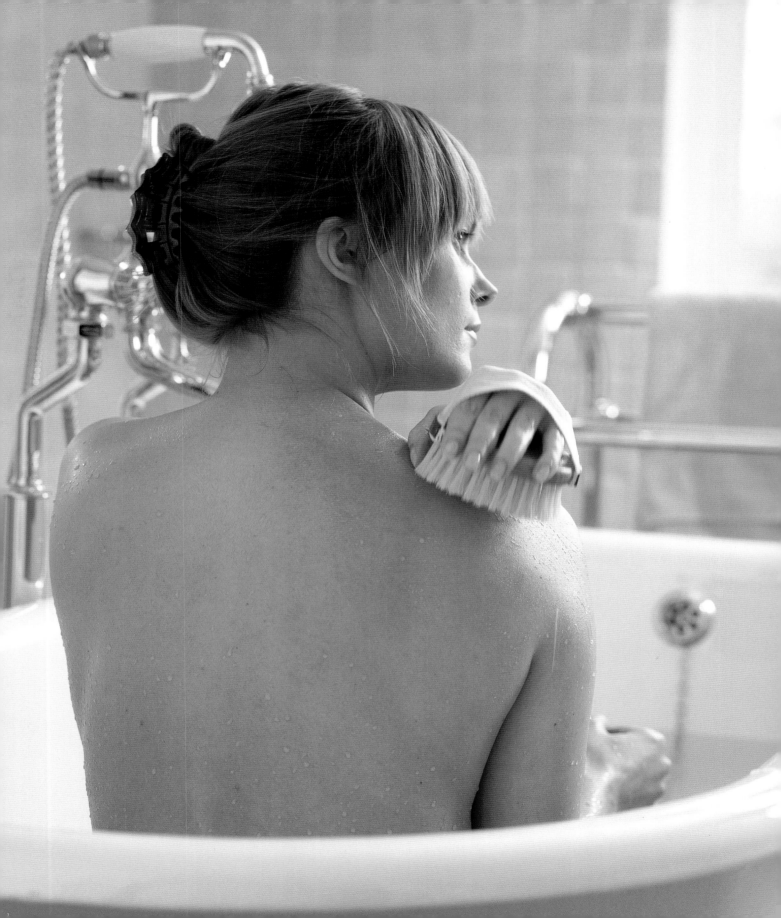

MIDDAY RESCUES

This is the time when aromatherapy oils can make the difference between a wasted afternoon and a productive one. A few drops of an energizing citrus oil such as lemon, lime, orange, mandarin, or bergamot on a handkerchief is all you need for a post-lunch pick-me-up (see pages 98–99 for more ideas).

If you find yourself stressed out, nervous, or angry, practice some alternate nostril breathing. By inhaling through one nostril and exhaling through the other, you'll balance your body and soothe your nervous system. Repeat the following at least five times or until your anxiety fades.

1 Close your right nostril with your right thumb and inhale deeply through your left nostril.

2 Hold for a few seconds, then close your left nostril with the middle finger of your right hand, release your thumb, and exhale through your right nostril.

3 Without moving your middle finger, inhale deeply through your right nostril.

4 Hold for a few seconds, close your right nostril with your thumb, and then release your left nostril before exhaling.

EVENING KICKBACKS

If you have trouble switching off after a hard day, literally scrub off your stress in the shower. Visualize your worries being washed down the drain as you go to work with your loofah or massage mitt. Change into some feel-good clothes (choose natural fibers such as cotton, linen, silk, wool, or cashmere) and you'll feel refreshed and ready for relaxation.

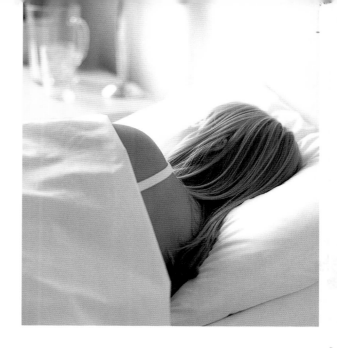

Slowing down at the end of a busy day is not being lazy, it's essential for a good night's sleep and to prepare yourself for the next day. Of course, some day's-end activities are more nurturing than others. Spending the evening flipping TV channels may feel relaxing, but if you try to sleep immediately afterward, your mind will still be busy and your body tense. Instead, set aside at least an hour before bedtime for some quiet pampering time.

Never end the day with a head full of unfinished tasks and chores. Rather than add to your neverending to-do list, change your perspective with a "done" list instead. Write down all the things you've achieved during the day and go to bed with a sense of achievement, not stress.

The best position to sleep in is on your side, as it encourages deep breathing through your nostrils, rather than the shallow breathing through your mouth (and snoring) you do when lying on your back. Most of us sleep with too many pillows, which can cause neck strain. Instead, use only one pillow and tuck it right into your neck to make sure your head and spine stay in alignment.

a quiet life

Silence is golden—and elusive. From the minute your alarm goes off, your head is filled with noise. Music blaring, people shouting, car alarms wailing, even your partner snoring. No wonder silence is so hard to find, which makes it all the more important to experience a few moments of tranquility every day.

It's hard to be productive with a racing mind, but when your mind's quiet, you can focus on what you're doing while still being able to see the whole picture. You can learn how to slow down and enjoy a state of internal silence by practicing the following techniques.

MEDITATION simply means concentrating on a mantra to replace your normal internal chatter while breathing deeply. This replaces stress with deep relaxation. Long-term benefits include clear thinking plus greater tolerance and decreased irritability, which not surprisingly leads to improved relationships and a feeling of happiness and well-being. The technique involves sitting comfortably (on the sofa, in a park, or even on a train) for 15–20 minutes with your eyes closed, silently repeating a mantra. Your breathing slows down as your mind experiences an inner silence while being wide awake. Bliss? Not far from it. For the first few times, choose a quiet place where you won't be interrupted (unplug the phone) and turn down the lights/close the blinds. Make sure you're comfortable and then start to imagine each part of your body relaxing. Begin with your scalp and work down to your toes, all the while thinking a two-syllable mantra (anything works: try "feel-good," "re-lax," or "me-time"). Concentrate on your breathing, and when thoughts break through the calm just let them come and go.

After 15 minutes, open your eyes and sit quietly for a few minutes before getting up and on with your day.

VISUALIZATION was devised by a radiotherapist who became convinced that patients' minds could be used to heal their bodies. Studies show that visualization encourages activity in the right side of your brain, which produces positive thoughts and energy. All you need is your imagination. If you want to relax, simply visualize a place that you find calming and peaceful. It could be an open meadow or wide lake (nature automatically regenerates the heart), or somewhere you associate with happy times (a beach or even your childhood bedroom). Whatever you choose, picture the scene in detail—the color of the sea, the sound of the waves, the smell of suntan lotion, the feel of sand under your feet. Once you've built up a vivid picture, you'll be able to recreate it quickly in times of need. Visualization can also be used to promote good health (look inside yourself and imagine your internal organs smiling at you), or to calm apprehensive thoughts about the future (you can imagine yourself acting the part while knowing no harm will come to you). However you use it, visualization works like a mini mind vacation. Simply find somewhere quiet to sit comfortably, be aware of your posture and breathing, and keep your feet on the ground to feel centered during your head trip.

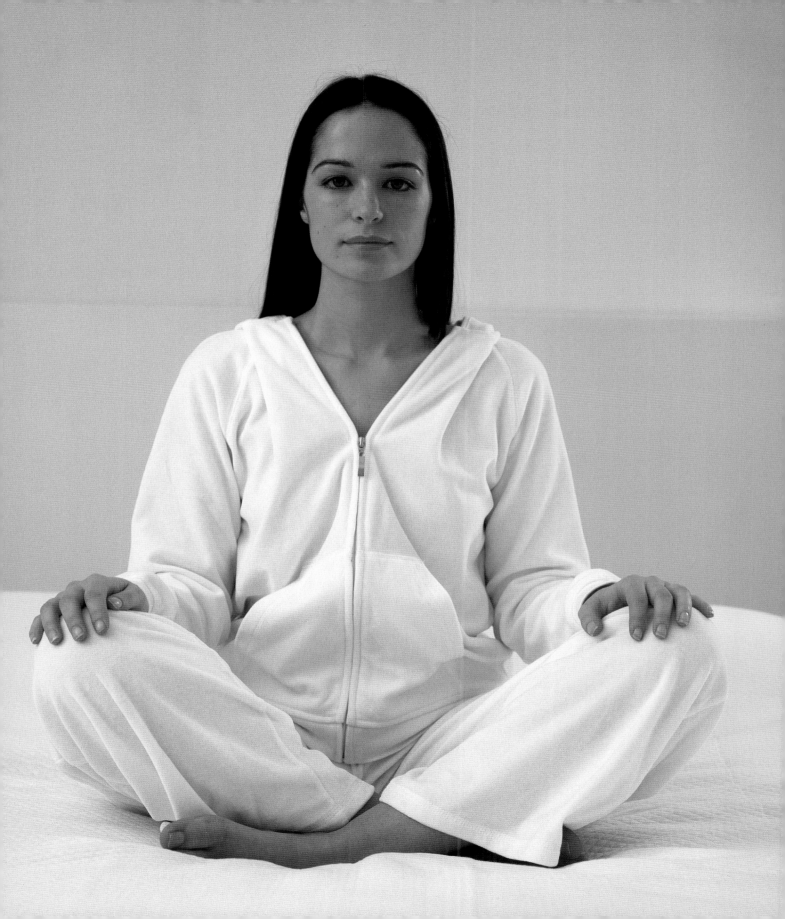

stress strategies

In today's busy world, the following two mind games can
make all the difference between surviving and thriving.

ONE MINUTE THAT COULD SAVE YOUR DAY
You don't need 20 minutes to meditate. You can turn
a stressful situation into a one-minute mini-meditation.

I Terrified you're going to ruin your presentation?
Paranoid about office politics? Just sad for no reason?
Avoid your mind's doom-and-gloom spiral: "If I blow
this I'll lose my job," and so on. Take a deep slow breath
and observe *exactly* how you're thinking and feeling.

2 Now breathe out and put those observations
into words: "I'm scared because I haven't done enough
research," or "I messed up my last presentation—why
should this one be any different?"

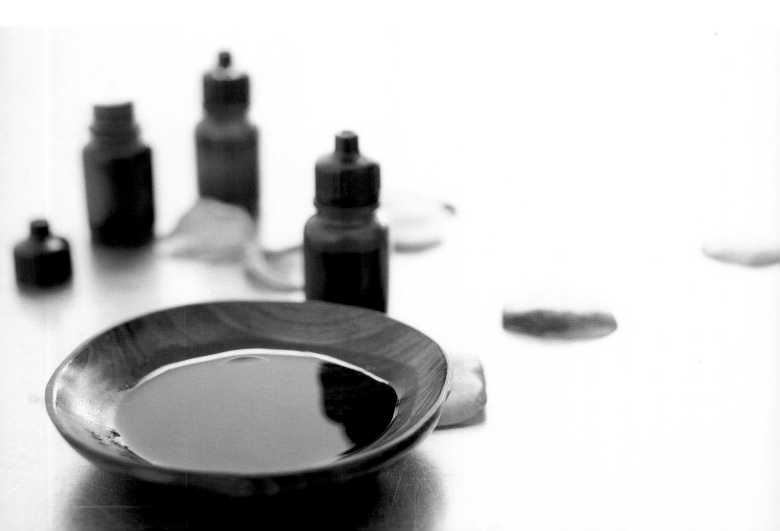

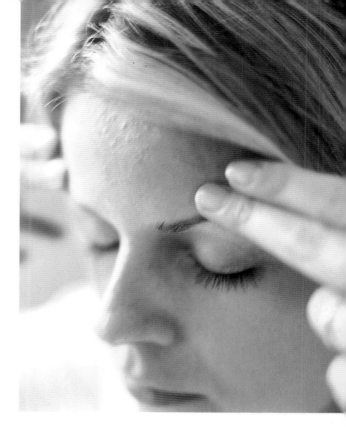

3 Keep breathing deeply as you put your fears into words. Simply by acknowledging exactly what's going on, you can do something practical or at the very least shift your perspective. Fear is simply an energy, and you can choose to use it to your advantage.

□ What can you find out in the next hour that will help you feel more confident? Who can help you with this last-minute research? What can you learn from this experience so you never let it happen again?

□ Maybe you're much better prepared than last time? Maybe you're more experienced? Perhaps your audience is less intimidating? Perhaps you know your subject better? Just looking at what else could be possible can change your mindset and make you feel so much more positive about the challenge ahead.

ONE SENTENCE THAT CAN SAVE YOUR SANITY

The word *mantra* means "mind tool" in Sanskrit, and the right one can stop the most stressed mind in its tracks. You already have many mantras in your head, and you're probably not even aware of them.

□ "I always ruin things."
□ "I can't be alone."
□ "It never works out for me."

Your brain works by repetition, so the longer a thought stays there, the stronger it will be. No surprise, then, that eventually that thought becomes an automatic reaction every time you hit hard times. Guess what? If you think it never works out for you, it rarely will.

So what could you invent to replace that self-defeating phrase? You want to make a concrete contradiction, not just an airy positive platitude.

So "It never works out for me" can't be replaced with a Pollyanna-ish "Life is wonderful"—your mind's too smart for that. Far more powerful is a mantra that can be supported with hard evidence. "I will survive, I always do" puts you in control, if not of what happens in your life, then at least of how you deal with it. Next, write down the evidence to back it up—all the times when things didn't go your way, but you got through it and came out the other side a stronger person.

INSPIRATION TO INVENT YOUR OWN MANTRA

□ "If I'm facing in the right direction, all I have to do is just keep going."
□ "I know no matter how bad this feels, it will pass."
□ "What doesn't kill me makes me stronger."
□ "There is always a solution."

The next time life speeds up, repeat your chosen phrase in your head. You may be surprised by how much quicker your panicky mind slows down again.

indulge your senses

When you're busy, it's easy to forget there's more to you than just practical thoughts and actions. To nurture yourself completely, you have to get in touch with all your five pleasure senses.

These get forgotten in times of stress, when shallow breathing stops you from smelling what's around you, and eating on the run stops you from tasting fully what you put in your mouth. But sensory deprivation is one route to madness, so it's no wonder that fully indulging your senses feels so relaxing.

What gives you pleasure is unique, so start off by making a list of what you love.

I LOVE…
I love the taste of…
I love the smell of…
I love the sight of…
I love the sound of…
I love the touch of…

Stress stops us from appreciating the simple things in life, so it may take a while to come up with more than the obvious. You'll probably be quick to write "chocolate cake" down under taste, but you need to go deeper to find your true sensory pleasures. Perhaps the taste of your child's skin? Or your partner as you kiss him goodnight? Feeding yourself foods that make you feel good (rather than uncomfortable and bloated) is a treat for your taste buds as well as your body. And making meals a pleasure by eating slowly will indulge your senses far more than shoveling food down at your desk. Read on for more inspiration.

SMELL
Surround yourself with scents that calm you down or lift you up, depending on what you need. Burn essential oils at your desk, or sprinkle them in your bath water or on your pillow at night (turn to pages 98–99 for more ideas). Take a trip around a perfume department and hunt out scents that bring back happy memories. Perhaps there's one that reminds you of your teenage party years, or a brand your mother used when you were young. Wearing them now will have an instant effect on your mood, whether it's giving you that excited feeling before a night out or making you feel safe and secure.

SIGHT
Do your surroundings please you? When was the last time you really noticed what you live with every day? Perhaps your bedroom needs painting, or the curtains in your living room are threadbare. If your workplace is a depressing sight first thing in the morning, take in photos from home or buy a plant for your desk. If you spend your days in an office, get out into green spaces at lunchtime for an instant feel-good effect.

SOUND
What music gives you a warm feeling? Dig out your old records and make up compilations to play in your car. And it's not just music that soothes us. Does the sound of a particular friend's voice make you feel

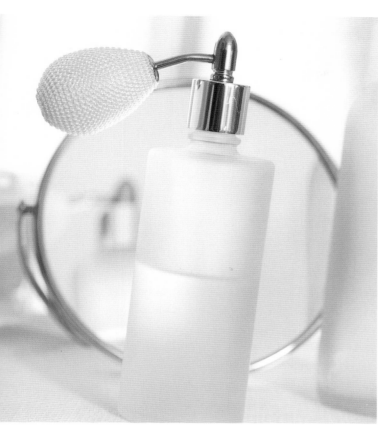

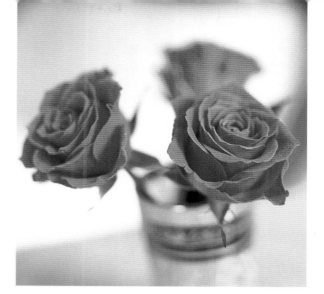

supported? Would the tinkling of a wind chime on your porch relax you (or drive you and your neighbors mad)? The sounds of nature are always soothing, so invest in a CD of water, waves, or wind rustling through the trees to play after a hard day.

TOUCH

Do the clothes you wear feel great against your skin, or do they have scratchy seams and uncomfortable zippers? Do you sleep on good-quality cotton sheets, or rough old polyester ones? Do you take the time to massage body lotion into your skin after bathing or just rub yourself down with a rough towel? Do you give yourself (or someone else) a hug every day? Many of us are desperately touch-deprived, so let your friends and family know you care by regularly showing them affection.

Include as many sensory pleasures in your day as possible, particularly when you're scared, sad, or bored. Wear your favorite perfume to the dentist, or a cashmere sweater when visiting your difficult mother-in-law. You'll enjoy every moment just a little bit more.

mood improvers

Our bodies are set up for happiness. We get a natural rush of endorphins (feel-good chemical messengers) when laughing, doing physical exercise, being with people we love, or feeling completely relaxed. But we can manufacture the same response by *remembering* an experience that recreates positive emotions.

MAKE YOUR OWN ENDORPHINS

It's easy. Start off relaxed and just think of a happy thought: your partner doing something special for you, your friend showing how much she cared. Then make this thought more and more vivid in your mind until you begin feeling the good vibes you experienced when it took place. Indulge in the sensation until you become aware of which parts of your body feel good. Do you have a tingle in your stomach or a warm glow in your heart? Hold that feeling and really pay attention to it. You want to be able to conjure up the same sensation again and again, particularly when what's going on around you may not be so positive.

Go all Julie Andrews and make a list of your favorite things. These can be things people have said to you or done for you, or simple pleasures such as stroking your cat. Now you have a list of the happy thoughts and memories that you can call on when you want to experience an endorphin rush any time, anywhere.

SPONTANEOUS SMILE INDUCERS

Smiling is a very serious business—it releases tension and promotes a feeling of total well-being.

For a few days, observe what makes you smile spontaneously. We're talking a genuine smile, not the socially acceptable one you put on when meeting someone new. A genuine smile lifts your spirits. What events, situations, and people produce your inner (and perhaps outer) smile? Make a note of every smile sighting until you have a list of spontaneous smile inducers. Then treat yourself to at least two a day. Remember: these are things that make you feel good, not things you think *should* make you feel good. If the very thought of going to the gym makes you smile, put it on your list. If not, it's never going to be one of your spontaneous smilers—however much you want it to be.

PRACTICE YOUR OWN INNER SMILE

As an alternative to endorphin-fueled mood improvers, you can recreate a smiley feeling with an inner smile.

1 Start by sitting comfortably. You can do this anywhere—on the bus, at work, or stuck in traffic.
2 Allow a smile to come into your eyes. Then let it spread to the rest of your face so the corners of your mouth turn up slightly.
3 Now smile into any part of your body that's tense and feel it begin to relax.
4 Next, smile into any part of your body that feels good and thank it for keeping you healthy.
5 Last, smile into the parts of your life that are working and allow yourself to feel grateful—for a work project that's going well, a nurturing friendship, or a home that makes you feel relaxed and secure.

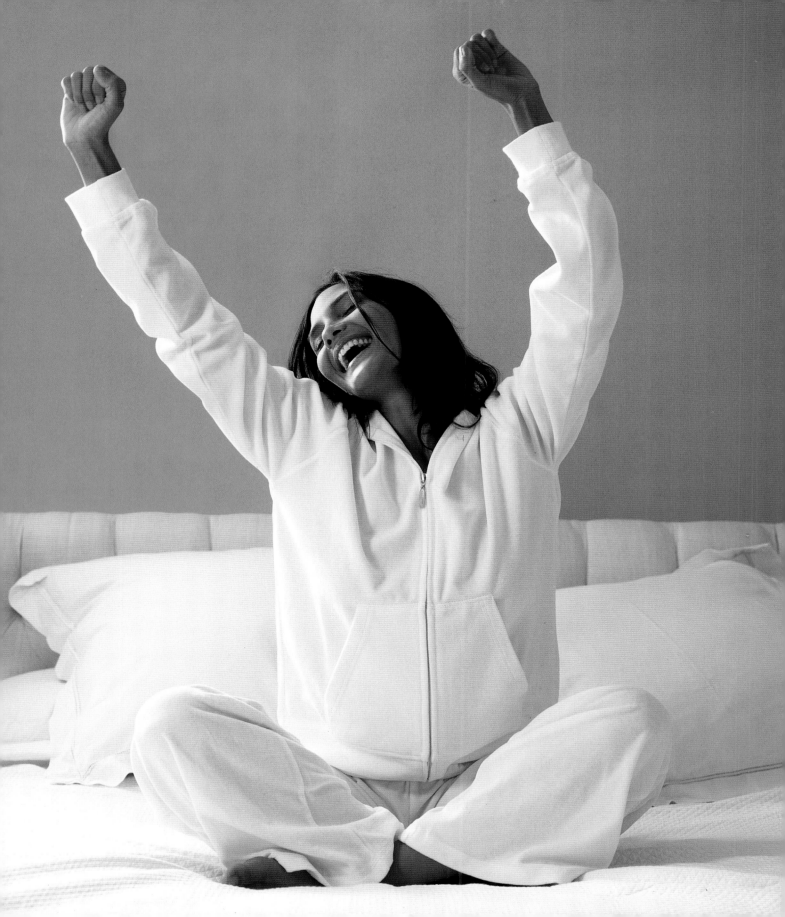

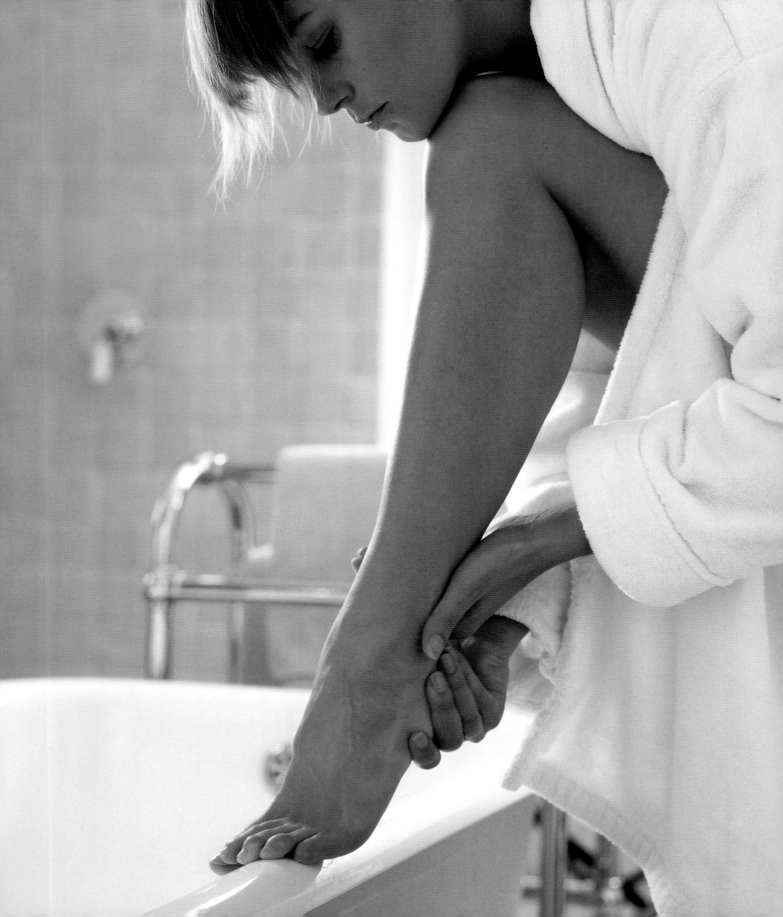

20 instant rescue remedies

For when you're *feeling* less than your best.

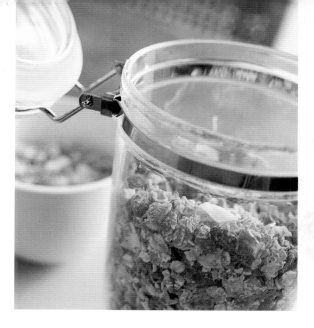

I   Sore, tired feet love a warm foot bath with either a handful of epsom salts or five drops of peppermint essential oil added. Finish with a shot of cold water from the shower to reduce any puffiness before drying thoroughly.

2   When you hit a tired spell, ditch the coffee and instead drink two glasses of pure water quickly. Follow with a ten-minute walk outside, which will stimulate your heart, lungs, muscles, and mind.

3   Alcohol lowers your body's supply of vitamins B and C, so rather than drinking water the morning after make yourself a juice for a far more potent hangover cure. Top marks go to a carrot or celery and apple combination, which will help rebalance your body. And give yourself a better chance of recovery by taking the detoxing herb milk thistle before and after drinking. It works by helping your liver process alcohol, so reducing the effects of any hangover the next day.

4   When times are tough, it's even more important to connect with the people you love. So no matter how busy you are, make time to see and speak to those closest to you. Knowing you are cared about puts even the worst day into perspective.

5   If your skin's prone to flushing in hot atmospheres, drink a cup of hot peppermint tea, which will instantly cool down your system.

6   Don't even think about starting the day with a bagel or white toast (both refined carbohydrates) when you're feeling less than energetic. What you need are complex carbs (preferably uncooked ones) such as granola, with a bit of protein for slow, sustained energy throughout the day.

7   To override a midday or mid-afternoon energy slump, eat a slice of avocado on whole-wheat toast or a small handful of nuts or seeds for a steady, long-lasting high.

8   New ideas come from a fresh mind, so when you're stuck, take a break for five minutes or longer. Gaze out of the window and let your mind wander, or go for a walk and let the fresh air blow through your brain. By the time you return, you'll be thinking far more calmly and clearly.

9   Release the tension in a tight, stressed jaw by biting into a crunchy apple. Apples are also the perfect way to freshen breath on the go, as they cause your mouth to step up saliva production, breaking down food particles that may be causing bad breath.

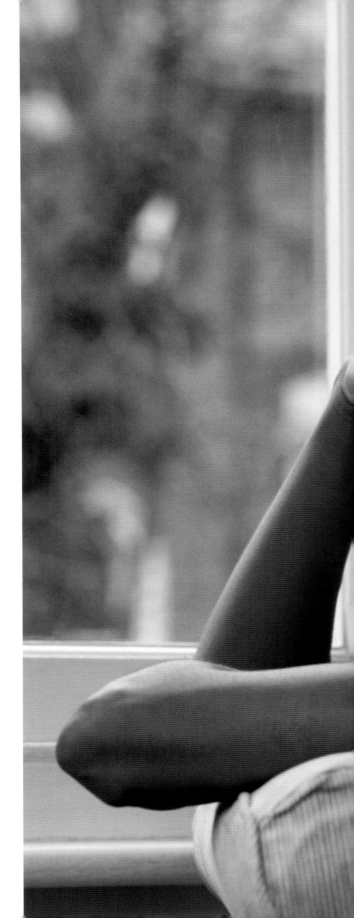

IO When you have trouble sleeping, eat a small portion of starchy food such as a piece of whole-wheat bread with fruit preserves before bedtime. But avoid butter or margarine, as fat will interfere with the sedative effect.

II For a quick energy boost, grate a small spoonful of fresh ginger into a mug of hot water. The same mixture can also be used as a hot compress for lower back ache. Dip a washcloth in the water, wring out, and hold over the problem area (avoid if you're pregnant).

I2 Ease winter cold and cough symptoms with a cup of parsley tea. Boil one bunch of parsley in a small saucepan of water, pour the mixture into a cup, and drink before you eat. You can also soothe congestion by massaging your chest with five drops of eucalyptus oil mixed with one tablespoon of vegetable oil.

I3 Never wait until you feel lousy to take echinacea. The time to start is when you first feel you're coming down with something. And don't be tempted to take it long term, as studies show that echinacea loses its immunity-boosting powers if your body gets too accustomed on the effects.

I4 Tell yourself you'll have a good day and you probably will. Research shows that people who think good things will happen to them are usually right, so next time your mind takes a negative turn, ask yourself what more positive outcome could be possible. We make our own thoughts, so we may as well make them optimistic.

I5 If a busy mind is waking you at 2A.M., keep a notebook by your bed and write down any problems, insights, or solutions. With your head clear you'll be much more likely to fall straight back to sleep, and you can deal with things far better in the morning.

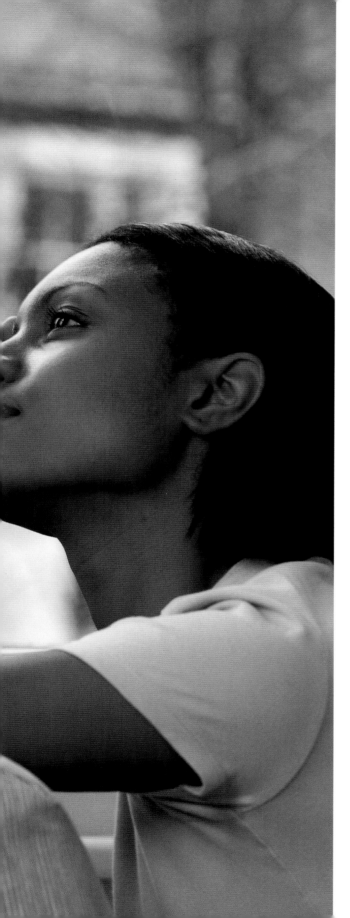

16 When you're feeling low in energy, eat foods rich in vitamin B, which is required for the production of energy. These include fruit, vegetables, seeds, nuts, whole grains, and fish. Bananas are also a great energy boost due to their high concentration of natural sugar, which produces a slow, steady shot in the arm. And rather than three large meals a day, eat smaller meals more often to sustain you.

17 Tense, stressed headache? Gently press your first two fingers just under the bone at the base of your skull either side of your spine. Lean back onto your fingers and then work in gentle circular movements down each side of your neck, spending a little longer on tender areas.

18 Another headache cure. Soak your feet for ten minutes in a bowl of warm water mixed with a teaspoon of cayenne pepper, as the heat will draw blood away from your head and ease the pain. Foods that heal headaches are salty, so try eating a couple of olives in brine. If after a few minutes this doesn't help, quickly drink two glasses of cool water.

19 Book your next time off from work, even if you're not going away on vacation. Just knowing you will have time to relax then will help you to keep going when life feels out of control. Even if you've only managed to clear one day, plan to do something you'll really enjoy—no chores allowed.

20 Determine what parts of your day make you the most stressed (for example, sitting in traffic, doing housework, answering e-mails), and then work out a way to lessen your irritation (solutions could be listening to books on tape, getting a cleaner, only responding to mail that really needs a reply).

ten ways to look after yourself when you're busy

I GIVE YOURSELF THE FIRST TEN PERCENT
You can only look after others if you first take care of yourself properly.

2 INVEST IN YOURSELF
Whether that means me-time, great-quality food, or new experiences.

3 TAKE THE PHONE OFF THE HOOK AFTER DINNER
You don't have to be available to others 24 hours a day, seven days a week.

4 GET A GOOD NIGHT'S SLEEP
The average adult needs eight hours' sleep a day, so improve your chances of deep rest with a good-quality mattress and pillows.

5 SURROUND YOURSELF WITH "UP" PEOPLE
Your environment has a profound effect on you, so make sure the people you spend most time with are supportive.

6 PRACTICE DO-ANYWHERE DE-STRESS STRATEGIES
For example, take three deep breaths while rubbing the insides of your palms to improve blood supply and stimulate circulation.

7 ONLY DO ONE THING AT A TIME
It's OK to do two things at once, but only as long as you don't need to do either of them very well.

8 KEEP THINGS IN PERSPECTIVE
In times of stress, it's important to stop and admit that what you're facing is actually more annoying than life-threatening.

9 HAVE A SENSE OF HUMOR
Laughter reduces stress hormone levels, so find something to lighten your mood every day.

IO DO WHAT MEANS THE MOST TO YOU
Figure out what brings you the most joy and make it your mission to find time for that every day of your life.

last word

If you want to see what your thoughts were like yesterday, look at your body today. If you want to see what your body will be like tomorrow, look at your thoughts today.

OLD INDIAN SAYING

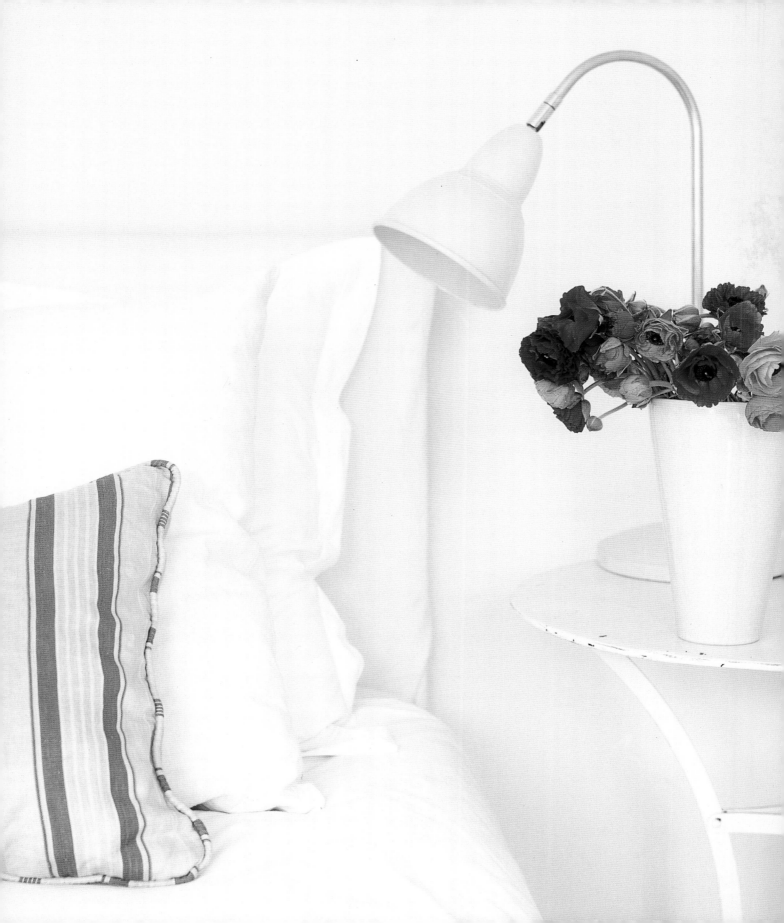

useful addresses

RETAILERS

Aveda
866 823 1425
for stores
www.aveda.com

Barneys New York
660 Madison Avenue
New York NY 10021
212 826 8900
www.barneys.com

Bath & Body Works
800 395 1001 for stores
www.bathandbody
    works.com

Crabtree & Evelyn
800 272 2873 for stores
www.crabtree-evelyn.com

Crate & Barrel
650 Madison Avenue
New York, NY 10022
800 967 6696 for stores
www.crateandbarrel.com

**Giorgio Armani
Cosmetics**
www.giorgioarmani.com

Green People
www.greenpeople.co.uk

Laura Mercier Cosmetics
www.lauramercier.com

Origins
www.origins.com

Sephora
2103 Broadway
New York, NY 10023
212 362 1500
www.sephora.com

INFORMATION

**American Massage
Therapy Association**
500 Davis Street,
Suite 900
Evanston, IL 60201
847 864 0123
www.amtamassage.org
Help with finding a
massage therapist
near you.

**National Acupuncture and
Oriental Medicine Alliance**
6405 43rd Avenue Ct.
NW, Suite B
Gig Harbor, WA 98335
253 851 6896
www.acuall.org

Information on
complementary and
alternative medicine
and on finding a
practitioner near you.

**National Women's Health
Resource Center**
157 Broad Street,
Suite 315
Red Bank, NJ 07701
877 986 9472
www.healthywomen.org
Information resource
designed to encourage
women to pursue healthy
lifestyles.

OTHER RESOURCES

Calmia
52–54 Marylebone
High Street
London W1U 5HR
+44 845 0092450
www.calmia.com
Holistic lifestyle store and
inner beauty day spa.

Chelsea Nail Studio
5 Pond Place
London SW3 6QR
+44 20 7225 3889

Method Putkisto Institute
56 Derby Road
London SW14 7DP
To order the Method
Putkisto Face School
video, DVD, or manual
call +44 20 8878 7384
www.methodputkisto.com
See pages 26–27.

Phytomer
Call +44 1753 856836
for stockists and
mail order
www.phytomer.com
Sea water and seaweed
products.

Also available from
The Beauty Room
www.thebeautyroom.com

Pure Massage
3–5 Vanston Place
London SW6 1AY
+44 20 7381 8100
www.puremassage.uk.com
Body and face massages,
also Introduction to
Massage Course.

index

acknowledgments

Many thanks to The Method Putkisto Face School (see pages 26–27); Tracy Hemmings at Calmia Inner Beauty Day Spa, who devised the de-stress facial (page 30) and facelift facial (page 36); Virginie Espil at Laura Mercier, Harrods, and Sheila Toofaneeram at Giorgio Armani, Harvey Nichols, London (see pages 48–49); Robyn Opie at the Chelsea Nail Studio (see pages 68–71); and Beata Aleksandrowicz at Pure Massage (see pages 84–87).

The author would like to thank all her wonderful friends and family.
Visit Liz Wilde's website at www.wildelifecoaching.com for information about her online programs, one-to-one coaching, and to subscribe to her free Monthly Motivator Mail.

picture credits

Photography by Daniel Farmer unless otherwise stated.
a=above, b=below, r=right, l=left, c=center

Page 14 © The Color Wheel Company (www.colorwheelco.com); **David Montgomery** endpapers, 23al, 24, 30al inset & background, 36–37l, 40–41, 49 background, 53, 59, 61c & b, 73, 98–99, 102, 112, 114–115l & ar, 119, 124–127; **Dan Duchars** 3, 30r inset, 44–45, 51, 62, 75r, 79 inset, 107, 109, 113; **Alan Williams** 4–5 / Alannah Weston's house in London designed by Stickland Coombe Architecture; **Jan Baldwin** 13 / Angela and David Coxon's family home in Kent, 61a, 80 / the Meiré family home, designed by Marc Meiré; **Debi Treloar** 15ar, 21, 57, 63, 105bl & r; **Chris Everard** 18–20, 75c, 81, 92; **Nicky Dowey** 22 & 23bl; **Martin Brigdale** 23ar; **William Lingwood** 23br; **Andrew Wood** 60, 75l; **Ian Wallace** 74r; **Tom Leighton** 79 background, 115br; **Simon Upton** 105al; **Polly Wreford** 123, 128.

Stickland Coombe Architecture 258 Lavender Hill, London SW11 1LJ, UK t. +44 20 7924 1699 www.sticklandandcoombe.com Pages 4–5
Angela Southwell Interior Design t. +44 1732 763246 angsouthwell@hotmail.com Page 13
Also featured in this home: Maybury tropical rustic furniture and accessories (www.mayburydesign.co.uk)

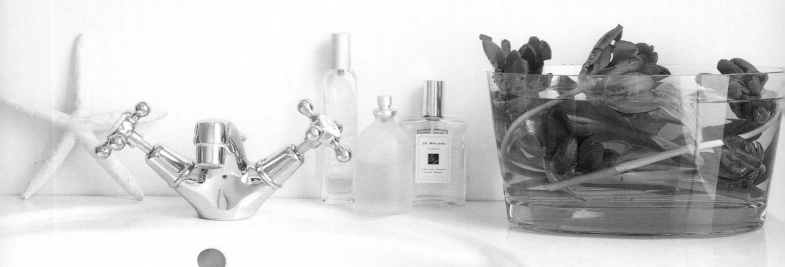

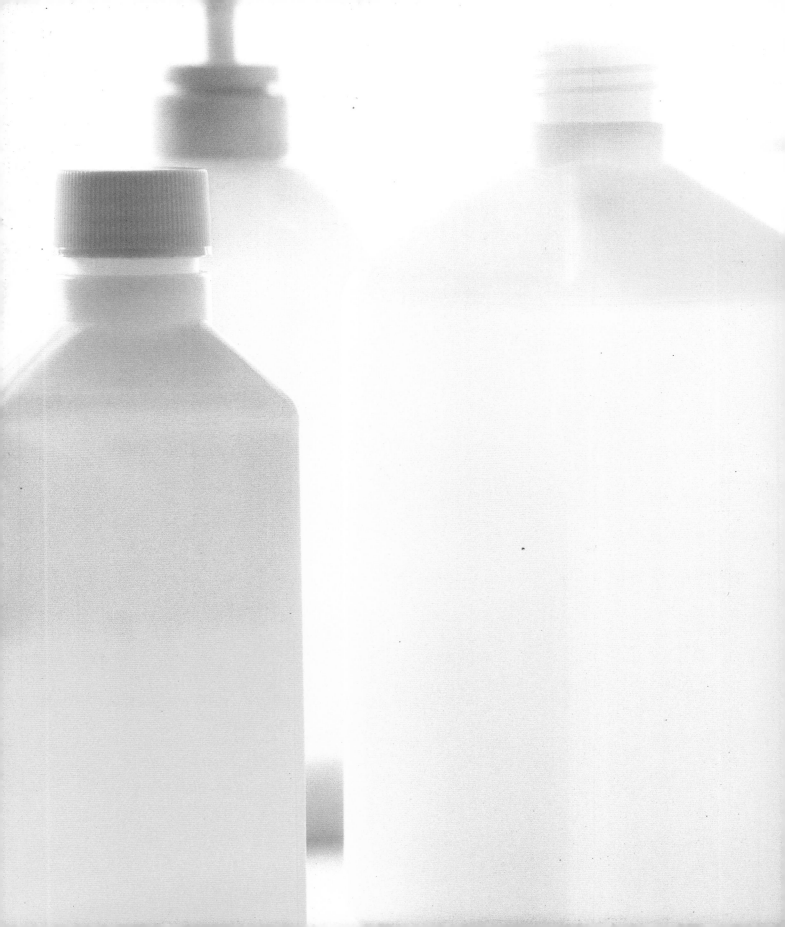